THE
METABOLISM
SOLUTION

THE
METABOLISM
SOLUTION

LISA LYNN

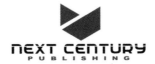

NEXT CENTURY
PUBLISHING

The Metabolism Solution
Copyright © 2015 by Lisa Lynn
The Metabolism Solution
Lose 1 Pound Per Day and Melt Belly Fat Fast

by Lisa Lynn
2nd Edition

Printed in the United States of America

ISBN 978-1-68102-010-5
Library of Congress Control Number: 2015901552

To contact Lisa Lynn for media appearances, book signings or speaking engagements:

Lisa Lynn
lisa@lynfit.com
203-295-8878
www.LynFit.com
LynFit Nutrition

Dedicated to all who have struggled with their weight, trying diet after diet, fasting, even starving themselves, as well as over-exercising, only to gain even more weight. It is my personal mission to help you lose weight and keep it off for life. *The Metabolism Solution* will radically transform your whole life, not just your body. You'll live a happier, healthier, and leaner life—so you can do what God sent you here to do.

With Deep, Heartfelt Gratitude

It's fitting that this book is called *The Metabolism Solution* because it truly contains the solution to all of your weight loss problems. My intention in writing it is to pass on what I've learned through my own struggles and studies as well as to pass on the blessings I've received.

All of the glory goes to God, as He is my strength and inspiration. I want to thank Him for giving me this opportunity to help so many people. As always, He guided me through the entire process.

Many thanks to Ken Dunn and the entire NCP team for all you've done. Rod Larrivee and Simon Presland, your attention to detail are greatly appreciated, and you've created a superb book.

Frankie, an angel sent from above, for putting it all together; and to my support team/prayer warriors (you know who you are) for sharing my passion and, most of all, for inspiring me to reach further and share more of myself in order to help others succeed. I could not have done it without your support and prayers.

Thank you, Mom and Dad, for giving me life. Thanks especially to you, Mom, for being my best cheerleader and picking me up every time I fell down.

Thank you, Jeff, for being such a loving husband even when I didn't deserve it and for loving me no matter what—especially through the darkest hours of my food withdrawal and endless hours of overwork following my life's mission. I couldn't have done it without you.

Thank you, Kiana and Kyle. I cherish you; your love, joy, and happiness brighten my life, and I am grateful for you. You make every day full of life, and you always provide me with great food content, not to mention always being good sports about eating your vegetables.

I am extremely grateful to and thank God for my best friends, my dogs, who sat with me at my feet every minute of every day as I wrote this book and provided me with unconditional love and constant kisses.

Thank you, Grandma and Grandpa, for teaching me how to cook delicious-tasting food and showing me that, yes, food is love.

I'm grateful also to the ministry at Faith Church, particularly Pastor Frank, who always knows how to keep my passion in line with God's Word and inspires me to keep fighting the good fight. Nothing is greater than our God, and any battle we face is no match for God's grace.

Loads of gratitude go to all of the supporters—all of you who have selflessly shared your stories with me. You inspired me to write this book. Each and every one of you touches me more than you know.

I am grateful to my physical body for carrying me through life and for staying strong and healthy, which allowed me to work on my mission every single day; and I never take that for granted.

Finally I'd like to thank my Grandmother Mary Fabrizio, whose courageous battle with pancreatic cancer sparked and fueled my passion and commitment to health and weight loss, and my Grandmother Hannah Smith, who struggled with diabetes and ultimately lost her leg from diabetes complications but never let it slow her down.

Stay Strong, Live Fearlessly, and Be Blessed with Vibrant Health!

THE

METABOLISM

SOLUTION

TABLE OF CONTENTS

ONE

How I Made Myself Fat and What I Learned

Few struggles frustrate us more than the struggle with weight loss. I know. I'm a recovering compulsive overeater and have struggled with food cravings since childhood. I grew up the child of two alcoholics, who themselves came from generations of addicts (specifically, but not limited to, alcoholism). Looking back at my life now, I feel I was born physically damaged, which left me anxious and prone to depression and faulty thinking. Most importantly, I felt spiritually void.

When I think of those very early years, I remember three things very clearly: feeling lonely, feeling unloved, and feeling unsafe. As an adult, I can see that my poor parents struggled so badly with their own addictions, just trying to stay alive, that they had nothing left to give me. Subsequently, as a child, I

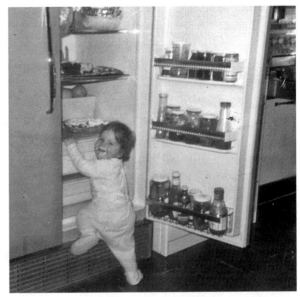

Food and I go way back

was left to parent myself. Growing up with an alcoholic father meant I always had to compete with the bottle, leaving me feeling like I wasn't good enough or worthy of his love. To this day, I still struggle with not feeling good enough.

It could have been worse, however. At least I had a roof over my head and no unexplainable bruises; but it was still bad. The emotional lessons I took from my childhood were more devastating than I ever realized at the time. I became the good survivor, the "I'll do it myself" girl, from an early age. Even when I didn't know how to take care of myself, I managed. I hid the fear and my feelings of unworthiness. I learned how to smile all the time, even while dying on the inside, and kept up this pretense well into adulthood.

It was only thanks to my mom's decision to get sober (over 40 years ago) following a 12-step program that I had my first inkling of hope. In her newfound sobriety, she decided to send me to a private Christian school. This was no easy feat as we were just about flat broke. It was there that I truly felt God's love for the first time. I felt safe, fulfilled, and whole.

17

When I was a child, food was my reward, my comfort, and my savior. I made the seemingly innocent decision to eat to appease my feelings of anger, frustration, and longing to cover up how uncomfortable I was inside—physically, emotionally, and spiritually. My childhood quick fix of overeating created a long-term problem. I became overly self-reliant and did not trust God's love and healing. I had food, and I had myself. I learned how to feed my hungry heart to numb painful feelings instead of dealing with them head on. Food was my drug of choice.

As an adult, I look back on those painful memories and realize that those childhood experiences, as horrible as they were at the time, shaped me into who I am today. It is only through experience that you grow into the awesome spiritual being God intends you to be. This process, this realization, takes time. With God's help, you can overcome anything no matter how big it may seem at the time. Nothing is bigger than our God. God was not the center of my life initially, and He certainly wasn't the center of my parents' lives during their alcoholic days. If food, alcohol, exercise—any addiction—becomes the center of your world, you are in trouble. In my own spiritual healing, I've learned to forgive myself and others, as well as to have faith. There is a direct correlation between physical fitness and spiritual fitness.

My father died a horrific death from lung cancer two years ago while still an active alcoholic and compulsive smoker. He left behind a legacy of alcoholism and addiction that still affects our family to this day. At the end, he was scared to die. Despite how badly he was suffering, he was afraid he wasn't forgiven. How well I remember our last conversation: "Daddy, you don't have to be brave for us, and you don't need to suffer anymore. Not only do we love you, but God loves you, and your sins have already been forgiven through His Son, Jesus. You can rest knowing that you are His child, and as long as you believe in Him and ask for forgiveness, your earthly suffering can transform into a heavenly celebration." The chaplain gave him his last rites, and he died peacefully the next morning.

While tragic and painful, this experience will always be one of my fondest memories of my dad. How joyful to know that I was able to bring him to the Lord in such a peaceful way. And to this day, I know that even through a lifetime of alcoholism, smoking, and all the ungodliness that followed, God still loved him, just as He does all of us today. He is constantly teaching us that every health and life issue we face, including weight loss, is physically, mentally, and spiritually rooted and that we must address all three aspects for true healing to take place. Through that pain, through that blackness, through that tragedy, God loves us.

How can my mental and spiritual struggles and mistakes help you? Well, thanks to my own battle with weight, I have learned the most successful method for fast and guaranteed weight loss. Believe me, I have studied and tried just about every weight loss program out there. None of them worked for me.

I became vegetarian, meticulously counted calories, religiously kept a food journal, and exercised until I couldn't raise my arm to hold a book—but I only gained weight.

If you are one of the lucky ones who have a fast metabolism and never crave the wrong food, stop reading now. If you're like me and struggle with a dead metabolism and have to work at losing weight, then this book will change your life forever. I don't say that lightly. If you want to lose weight by tomorrow, forget everything you've ever learned and start this plan today.

By this point, you may be wondering what makes *The Metabolism Solution* so different from all of the other healthy eating plans you've tried. The biggest difference? It has an uncommon approach. No guilting, no shaming, no scaring. All food is good food, and all exercise is better than none; but there is a method to it, a scientific approach, that leaves out the "opinions" that tend to trip you up. More of anything isn't better; better is better. Why waste your time on dieting and weight loss plans that tell you only what you want to hear? Why waste time on empty promises when you can get results fast?

I have been where you are. Me, a fitness expert. I used to think my clients would not want to hear that. But I was wrong. Not only do I have a slow metabolism due to hypothyroidism, but I love to eat. My struggle with weight was a losing battle until I learned the secret to boosting my metabolism. It is my personal mission to share what I have learned. But it's not just about losing, it's about gain, too. I want you to experience the anti-aging benefits and vibrant health and vitality that eating with purpose brings. I want to teach you *The Metabolism Solution* so you can keep the weight off for life.

You can do it. When your food is in order, your whole life will be in order. It's worth every ounce of effort you need to put into it. Living *The Metabolism Solution* has not just helped me lose weight; it has changed my body and helped me be happier. Yes, happier. No more do I wake up every day crying and feeling hopeless because I can't control my weight. By letting go of any anxious, negative thoughts and surrendering to the process, you too can lose one pound every day until you reach your goal. I guarantee that if you follow *The Metabolism Solution* and stick to it, it works 100 percent of the time. Know that you can live a life of vibrant health and vitality!

NOW IS THE TIME TO CHANGE YOUR LIFE FOREVER

Do you want to lose one pound a day? *The Metabolism Solution* is the way to get into the best shape of your life, guaranteed. It's as simple as just making a decision. Making the decision to change. Sounds so easy, doesn't it? When you decide that you're sick and tired of being sick and tired, then and only then are you ready to make the necessary changes needed to lose weight for life. Deciding—that's the first step.

My story began with excuses. Sound familiar? I thought that losing weight was for everyone else, but not me, the woman who helps thousands of people radically transform their own bodies fast. I thought that because of my hypothyroidism, which kept my metabolism at a snail's pace, I had to starve myself and work out like a crazy woman for hours every day, seven days a week (at the expense of a happier life—ironically, because I was trying to make myself happier and feel better by losing weight). I tried every diet from the Caveman's to South Beach to Atkins to high-carb to low-carb—you name it. I became a vegetarian for a while in a last-ditch attempt to control my growing weight. I would starve myself and then binge on all that I'd been missing. I even joined Overeaters Anonymous. And finally, I told myself that there was nothing more for me to do and I had to learn to accept myself the way I was. I received the same advice from a therapist: "Learn to love yourself the way you are." Could I forgive myself for not being a size six? Possibly. But I just didn't feel good physically. I was becoming depressed, sad, and desperate. I couldn't even hear God's voice because the self-imposed negative nagging in my head was so loud.

Do you know what I mean? I hated seeing myself in the mirror, and frankly, I was sick and tired of being sick and tired. I fought with food; I struggled to change how I ate and instead became addicted to healthy foods like oatmeal and high-priced whole grains. The more I read and the more I heard about healthy eating for weight loss in the media, the more confused I became.

THE SCALE IS NOT YOUR GOD.

I soon lost all hope. I tried every supplement—even those that made my heart race at a frightening pace. I paid any price necessary to see any and all diet gurus about getting my body back on track. People came to me for this kind of knowledge and support, yet I couldn't help myself. That's what made it worse. I was a high-level master trainer, a highly regarded sports-nutrition specialist, and I couldn't help myself.

LEARNING FROM THE VERY BEST
Food and I go way back. My mother tells me how I couldn't be kept from the chocolate cake in the fridge at the age of two, as the photo in this chapter proves. My weight struggle started soon after. Yet I was somehow drawn to a healthy lifestyle. (I thank God for that. What would have happened to me otherwise?) To be brutally honest, I was obsessed with reading and learning everything I could about healthy and fit living because I was so unhappy inside.

Looking back, I truly believed that I was valued only because of the number I reached on the scale and the size I wore. I thought I would just be happier, fit in better, and be more successful if I could not pinch that inch on my stomach. It seemed so many of my friends could eat what they wanted and never gain an ounce. They were losing weight. I couldn't stand to look at myself

REPLACE FEAR WITH FAITH.

in the mirror. I felt hopeless, convinced that being fit and at a reasonable weight just wasn't for me. The irony was not lost on me that I was just starting out in the fitness business while going through my own personal fitness struggle. I studied everything I could get my hands on about losing weight, nutrition, and working out. At my heaviest I topped the scale at almost 50 pounds over where I wanted to be. I was helping others, but I couldn't help myself.

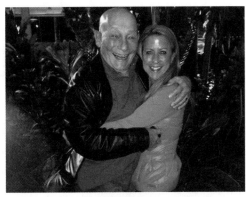

All smiles with Dr. Fred Hatfield

It wasn't until I was asked to work with Dr. Fred Hatfield, an internationally renowned fitness expert, founder of a fitness magazine that is now Men's Fitness, and the first person to lift over 1,000 pounds, that I finally had my Aha! moment. I was obsessively working out for three or more hours daily when Dr. Hatfield came into the gym in 1991 looking for trainers to work on a study he was running. The study would test the effectiveness of the American Heart Association's program combined with an extreme fat-loss program developed by a private company called Cybergenics versus Dr. Hatfield's own ICOPRO (Integrated Conditioning Systems) system. The former followed the AHA's food pyramid and added 30-minute calisthenics workouts three times a week. The latter used the ICOPRO system, also known as Thermic Force, which was a combination of scientific weight training, other types of training, psychological and nutritional strategies, the targeted use of supplements, and other techniques. At the time, I didn't realize that top fitness and nutrition experts, as well as elite athletes, turned to Dr. Hatfield for help. I had no idea who he was or that my life was about to change drastically.

I signed up to work with Dr. Hatfield, but I still clung to my doubts and fears. My mind told me that it would work for everyone but me. I thought I knew better; I was so naïve. How could eating more and exercising less (albeit in a more efficient way) cause such drastic changes in my body? No way. If starving myself and spending three hours at the gym wasn't making me leaner and fitter, how could less exercise possibly work?

Candidates in the study, both men and women, were not just overweight but also obese, with little to no knowledge about exercise and healthy eating. As I watched them finally be able to begin to change their bodies, it became obvious to me that everything I had been doing up to that point was all wrong. Everything I had learned about weight loss was fear-based. Fear of never being able to eat your favorite food. Fear of being judged. Fear of failure. I began to realize that dieting and exercising out of fear is no way to succeed.

For *The Metabolism Solution*, I took everything I learned from Dr. Hatfield and combined it with my own research and experience to finally get myself healthy. I cut down my gym time, focusing on better exercise instead of more reps. I discovered that specific foods could speed my weight loss, boost my metabolism, and that lean whey protein is necessary. I learned that a simpler plan is the more effective one and that smart, scientific supplements could truly make a difference without endangering my life. It was hard to make the change, but I am so glad I did.

MIRACLES COME FROM MOTIVATION

The most frequently asked question I get every day is about one of my appearances on The Dr. Oz Show when we discussed raspberry ketones. I've been on Dr. Oz's show repeatedly over the years to share fitness tips.

In this particular segment, Dr. Oz used two filled balloons to demonstrate how a supplement called raspberry ketones can shrink fat cells by affecting the levels of an important hormone called adiponectin and tricking our bodies into thinking like a thin person. He placed the balloons in nitrogen, and they shrank to a smaller size. Dr. Oz explained that raspberry ketones can do the same for fat cells and thus make them easier for our bodies to burn. I was there to corroborate the segment as an expert. Dr. Oz's producers (as well as those of other television shows) call on me when it comes to discussions on fat loss and supplements because they know that I have been studying this topic for 25 years and continue to do so. Through my ongoing studies, I have learned that supplements combined with a thermogenic (fat-burning) diet and metabolic-boosting exercises are the only way to get weight off fast. You cannot supplement away a bad diet.

One positive thing I have learned about myself is that I'm coachable. If I'm told to do something, I do it. I don't question or analyze; I just do it. And this brings me to the magnificent Martha Stewart.

One thing people do not know about Martha is that she has an incredible "can do" attitude. She never makes excuses. If she doesn't know how to do something, she learns then does it. That remarkable God-given ability got her to where she is today and has taught me that anything—and I do mean anything—is possible. Decide to do it and do the do.

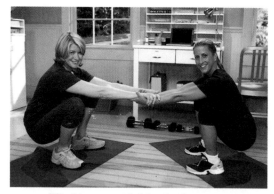

Working out with Martha Stewart

You might think it was at a high-end Pilates studio where I met Martha Stewart. You'd be wrong. I met Martha at a serious body builders' gym at 5:30 in the morning. That's the time when the "I Want Results" people work out; there's no socializing at that hour. I was working with a client who was a bathing suit model, and I would do my metabolic workout with him at the gym three to four days a week. Martha was there every morning on the treadmill. I was known around the gym as the trainer who got results—fast. She watched in amazement as I quickly morphed my client's physique into a lean, ready-for-the-beach (and camera) body. One day, when he was late for our appointment, Martha asked me for help.

I'll admit, I didn't know who she was. I could tell she was someone special because she had a presence about her. I probably would have been too nervous to speak with her if I had known who she was. Believe it or not, I said I couldn't help her that day because my client was on his way. But Martha didn't give up. The next day she asked me again, and this time I said yes.

I gave Martha the same speech I give all my new clients. Food impacts 80 percent of your results (unless you're over 40 and then it's 90 percent); exercise is only 20 percent (10 percent if you're over 40) of the equation to successful weight loss. I let Martha in on the weight loss secrets I had learned: to lose weight and fat fast, you need to boost your metabolism so you burn more calories all day long. The key? Drinking a whey protein shake every day within two hours of waking to boost your metabolism 25 percent, exercising better (and less), and eating the right kinds of foods.

After working with Martha for a bit, I learned that she had just gone through some difficult emotional times, had recently turned 40, and couldn't lose the weight "no matter what." Martha was frustrated that what she used to do no longer worked, and she was ready for change and results. She admitted that she had never had to watch what she ate; even during her days as a model, she always ate whatever she wanted. But she was learning what every wom-

> **IF MARTHA CAN, SO CAN YOU!**
>
> • **Have the right tools at your disposal— be it home or away.**
> • **Make fitness your first priority and start every day with a workout, no matter what.**

an learns: when you hit a certain age, what you did in your teens and twenties no longer works. Losing weight is just not that easy the older you get. To be honest, I believe it's harder for people who have never struggled with their weight to lose weight later in life—especially around the midsection—because they don't accept that they have to eat differently and work out differently in order to get their bodies to change.

Martha had tried several low-calorie diets and still couldn't lose the pounds she wanted to lose. Maybe you've been there? I explained that a whey protein shake would be better than starving in the mornings because it would tell her body to release fat from storage that could then be burned off as fuel. In contrast, just having coffee for breakfast told her body that food might not be coming so it should hold onto the fat to use for energy later.

She was eager to learn all I had to teach and constantly questioned me about everything. I convinced her to switch out the fattening foods and ingredients she ate for simpler ones, and she was stunned when the scale showed the pounds falling away. I explained how to use supplements safely to enhance and speed up the fat-burning process, help curb cravings, and block the unwanted carbs from being stored—a trick we all need at times. Lastly, I taught Martha how to work out specifically to boost her sluggish metabolism. I taught her everything I now teach you in these pages. In return, she called me the "only trainer who got results."

What I admire most about Martha is how incredibly strong, flexible, and unafraid of hard work she is. Her perseverance and determination to do whatever needs to be done is amazing. I have never met a busier person who still manages to get it all done. She prioritizes her fitness because she knows her health and wellness depend on it. It is at the top of her priority list—yes, even above cooking, scrapbooking, and entertaining. Home or away, Martha works out every day.

> **I WAS A GUEST on Martha's television show over 50 times. You can find many of these segments on YouTube. Among them I share exercise moves, and Martha and I prepare tasty and healthy foods—including the fish recipes in this book. I'll do whatever it takes to get people to exercise, and that includes cooking for Martha Stewart!**

We used to work out in the kitchen where she originally started her TV show or sometimes on her sun porch where she kept a huge flight cage of singing canaries. Her dogs would gather to watch, and occasionally one would give her a very wet face lick. Often one of her seven Himalayan cats would sit on top of her of while she did crunches. Why didn't I mind? The cat added resistance, which helps to strengthen, and it helped guarantee that Martha got her workout in a safe and comfortable environment in less time.

I see it firsthand all the time: those who work out at home get better results in less time because they are much more efficient and consistent since there is no travel to and from the gym. Even when Martha had houseguests, she would invite them to join us. She would never miss a workout with me. On Sundays I would meet Martha at her film studio to do cardio, and I would gather as many newspapers as I could, to get her to bike for hours if we weren't able to walk our local beaches.

TURN YOUR "I CAN'T" INTO "I CAN!"

Sometimes I had to bribe Martha with post-workout snacks to get her to finish exercising. I would blend a whey protein smoothie for her, which she drank from a champagne glass, naturally, or prepare an egg white breakfast (when a whey protein shake was on the menu for dinner) so she would finish every single exercise I had planned for the day. I'll do whatever it takes to get people to exercise, and that includes cooking for Martha Stewart.

The bottom line: You need a make-it-work attitude and the drive to do whatever it takes, for as long as it takes. You need to turn your "I can't" into "I can!" If Martha Stewart can do it, you can do it, too. I'm going to show you exactly HOW in the next chapter. Are you ready?

TWO

THERMOGENIC EATING FOR RADICAL WEIGHT LOSS

Every day I get emails from desperate people who have tried every diet on the planet and yet just can't seem to lose weight. Getting your body to switch over from fat-storing mode to fat-burning mode is easier than you think. Food is the problem and the answer. The solution is right in your refrigerator—or what's not in your refrigerator. So how do we get our bodies to switch from weight gain to weight loss while keeping our calorie intake high enough? By eating the right metabolism-boosting, thermogenic foods.

"Thermogenic" is an up-and-coming word in nutrition these days. It describes foods that take almost as many calories (or more) to digest as they put into the body. These foods increase your metabolism after you eat them.

Every single bite you put in your mouth counts and affects whether you gain or lose. Every bite. Even a small micro-dot of a bite has an effect on blood sugar, which is more sensitive than you can imagine. Before you put anything in your mouth, ask yourself, "Will this food enhance my metabolism or slow it down?" Eating only a "little" of a metabolism-slowing food will stop weight loss in its tracks.

The Metabolism Solution is all about super-charging your metabolism. Every food you eat or don't eat, every supplement you take, your metabolic workout—all provide a super-charge to your metabolism and get it burning like crazy so you can begin losing weight immediately. The more good choices you make daily, the faster you'll lose weight. Guaranteed!

Every time you eat chicken when you're supposed to have fish, skimp on the veggies, or don't drink enough water, you slow down your metabolism. If you eat protein that's high in fat like red meat, pork (it's not the other white meat), or processed meats such as sausage or bacon (yes, even turkey bacon), and the so-called healthy grains sold in gourmet markets, you are slowing down your metabolism. Just because a food may be good for you doesn't mean it's good for weight loss—especially if you have more than 10 pounds to lose.

What should you avoid then? Breads, rice, all pasta, chips, crackers, starchy vegetables like potatoes, butternut squash, oatmeal, and basically any food you don't see listed on my metabolic-boosting food lists that follow. Watch out for the diet-deceptor foods: avocados, nuts and oils (we eat too many), all nut butters, cheese, soy, almond and coconut milks, as well as all nondairy creamers (even the nonfat ones). These are usually the foods that keep you from losing weight in the first place. But don't worry—this book is full of delicious replacements for everything you crave. And in time, your cravings will stop, and you'll be leaner and feel better in no time at all.

The Metabolism Solution fixes these problems by rebooting your metabolism in a healthy way with wholesome, clean, fat-burning foods that supercharge your metabolism every time you eat them. And did I mention that these foods deliver powerful nutrients so you'll feel better fast? A clean food is one that is close to its natural state, not overly processed, not filled with loads of preservatives or added sugar, and without high levels of bad fats which include some saturated fats and all trans fats. What is a "clean" calorie? One that is free of saturated fats and derived from a natural source.

EVERYTHING YOU HAVE BEEN TAUGHT ABOUT EATING FOR WEIGHT LOSS IS ALL WRONG

When it comes to good nutrition, the one thing all experts agree on is that food is "The Holy Grail" of good health. The best way to get what you need is through your diet. But when it comes to boosting your metabolism, everything you have been taught is all wrong. Clean foods are great, but not all clean foods are *thermogenic*. I'll give you an example. Potatoes can be considered a clean food, yet they can slow weight loss due to the rise in your blood sugar. Other clean vegetables, like broccoli, increase your metabolism after you eat them.

Take carbohydrates as another example. Just because some carbs come from the earth doesn't mean they're good for metabolic boosting. I can hear you thinking: "But doesn't my body need carbs?" Yes it does, but not the kinds of carbs you're thinking about—breads, pastas, rice, and other whole grains. By and large, carbs are responsible for our nation's obesity issues. In fact, our bodies are now extremely resistant to weight loss and fat loss—specifically from the belly area—because we tend to overeat in this food group. If you want to eat a metabolic-boosting carb, pick a vegetable. In fact, the nutrients we need from carbohydrate sources can all be found in vegetables.

The same goes for foods labeled low-fat or nonfat. While they may be low in fat, they don't always give you that metabolic boost because they may spike blood sugar. In fact, most low-fat and nonfat foods are loaded with sugar. Not good for weight loss.

There are foods that you must avoid if you are trying to lose weight. To make it simple, I'm going to give you a list of what you can eat. If you don't see it on the lists, don't eat it. I urge you to memorize the lists so that you never succumb to food temptation. And remember, drinking a whey protein shake has you losing weight right away. One of its added benefits is that it helps you keep losing even while you learn (sometimes through trial and error) what you can and cannot eat when losing weight. Think of a shake as a little extra weight loss insurance.

The secret solution to boosting the metabolism is lowering blood sugar levels. Along with proteins and fats, carbohydrates are one of the three major components of food. Your body converts carbohydrates into glucose, which your cells burn for energy. Since glucose is transported to cells through your bloodstream, eating carbohydrates will cause your blood glucose level to increase. This is why it's crucial that you eat the kinds of carbs that won't spike blood sugar levels, such as vegetables. The good news? You can eat a lot more without spiking blood sugar! In addition, lowering blood sugar is the first priority when trying to get your body to shed fat. Why? Because blood sugar that isn't used by the body is turned into fat. That's right, fat. And we certainly don't need any additional fat storage when we are trying to lose weight and get fit.

That's why what you eat is 80 percent—nope, scratch that, more like 90 percent—of your weight loss success, especially if you're female and over 40 or have a damaged metabolism. What you don't eat makes all the difference. It's really not as simple as calories in and calories out, especially if you have a stubborn metabolism. If it were that simple, we would all simply eat what we want and count calories until we reach our daily limit. If you're reading this book, you've probably already tried that method with little success.

The Metabolism Solution is the healthiest diet of them all—it's the Ferrari of all plans; gluten-free, alka-linizing, low-carb, low-sugar, and low-fat. You cannot find a healthier and easier way to live. On my plan, I will not tell you that you can never ever eat a certain food again. You won't starve; you won't feel weak. You will eat.

LEAN, CLEAN PROTEIN

Protein is the foundation of *The Metabolism Solution*. It stabilizes blood sugar levels, which helps to curb cravings and feed your muscles, speeding up your metabolism. But I'm not talking any old protein—sirloin steak does not make the cut. The proteins eaten on *The Metabolism Solution* are chosen for their ability to elevate your metabolism. They have the right nutrients to do just that.

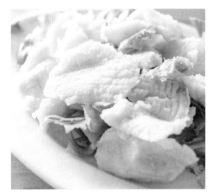

You may have seen me on Dr. Oz talking about specific fish—the types of fish that enhance metabolism. My line that gets quoted all the time is, "The lighter and whiter the fish, the better for your metabolism." Dr. Oz was in full agreement. White fish is lower in calories and extremely low in bad fat when compared to other,

The lighter and whiter your fish, the better for your metabolism

fattier fish like salmon and swordfish. While salmon and swordfish are not bad for you, a whiter fish is better. The whiter the fish, the faster you'll lose weight. Why? It's lower in calories and fat, making it very *thermogenic*. Stick to fattier fish (and poultry) one to two times a week, and make sure to weigh out your portions. Even an increase of one ounce can slow down your weight loss. If you find you're not losing at the pace you want, cut down even more on the fattier fish and switch to lighter, whiter fish.

THREE TO FOUR PROTEINS A DAY TAKE THE POUNDS AWAY

Whey Protein Shake (2 per day max.)	Shrimp 4 oz. (shelled)	Oysters 5 oz.
Whey Protein Bar (2 per day max.)	Sea Bass 4 oz.	Crab 4 oz.
	Snapper 4 oz. (all)	Lobster 1½ lbs. (whole)
Egg Whites (3 to 4)	Mussels 4 oz.	Calamari 4-5 oz.
Scrod/Cod 4 oz.	Chicken Breast 3 oz. (no skin)	Salmon 4 oz.
Flounder 4 oz.		Swordfish 4 oz.
Haddock 4 oz.	Tuna, Fresh or Canned 3 oz.	Sashimi 4 oz.
Halibut 4 oz.	Nonfat Cottage Cheese ½ cup	Sardines 3 oz.
Scallops 4 oz.		Herring 4 oz.
Orange Roughy 4 oz.	Mahi-Mahi 4 oz.	Trout/Rainbow Trout 4 oz.
Grouper 4 oz.	Clams 4 oz.	Turkey Breast 3 oz. (no skin)
Tilapia 4 oz.	Mussels 4 oz.	

Your best bet is to start your day with a quality whey protein shake for breakfast and try to eat fish once per day along with other sources of protein, such as egg whites. By varying your whey protein sources, you gain varied nutrient benefits while stimulating your metabolism.

Learn the list of proteins above, which are in order of their preference for weight loss. Remember, a serving is three to four ounces. Teens and men (sorry, ladies) can increase portions to four to five ounces each. Enjoy these baked, broiled, grilled, or steamed (without butter or skin). Aim for three to four servings per day unless noted. And if you find you're one of the lucky ones who loses weight fast, add an ounce to your portion.

THE RIGHT CARBOHYDRATES: SUPER VEGGIES FOR SUPER-FAST FAT LOSS

If you're like me and you like to eat a lot of food but need to keep your calories low in order to lose weight, vegetables are the key to your success. Don't like to eat your veggies? Keep trying different kinds and be sure to check out the recipes in this book. My vegetable recipes won't make you feel like you're denying yourself. The best thing about veggies (especially fibrous carbohydrates) is that they are nutrient-rich and will leave you full and satisfied because of their high fiber content. They support weight loss by decreasing your appetite and help to eliminate cravings for high-sugar foods. These good-for-you carbs slow down the digestive process, which helps rev up your metabolism.

Fiber, while not absorbed by your body, grabs fatty acids and other unwanted waste as it digests helping them, in turn, pass through your system. Think of fiber as a sponge that absorbs unwanted and unhealthy material while scouring your insides clean. Clean intestines let your body absorb more nutrients and vitamins, be they from diet or supplement. Constipation, a clogged system, feels horrible, so you must eat enough vegetables to insure adequate fiber. Another plus for these fibrous carb wonders: they speed your liver's cleansing process, which is important for optimal health, most especially when losing body fat.

> **WE ALL KNOW** that carbs such as bread, pasta, crackers, and of course all of the refined carbohydrates like cookies, cakes, and candies are not good for weight loss. BUT even the so-called "healthy grains" such as rice, oatmeal, potatoes, and any other carbohydrate (even if it's gourmet and found in a health food store) is not going to help you boost your metabolism. Keep it simple. Remember: If it's not found on the vegetable list, it's a starchy carbohydrate and will cause your insulin to spike and stop weight loss instantly ... even the tiniest of servings.

TEN VEGGIES A DAY MELT THE FAT AWAY

ALFALFA SPROUTS	COLLARD GREENS	RADISHES
ASPARAGUS	CUCUMBERS	SPINACH
BROCCOFLOWER	EGGPLANT	TOMATO JUICE (4 OZ.)
BROCCOLI	ESCAROLE	TOMATOES
BRUSSELS SPROUTS	GREEN BEANS	YELLOW BEANS
CABBAGE (ALL TYPES)	KALE	YELLOW SQUASH
CARROTS	LETTUCE (SERVING - 3 CUPS)	WAX BEANS
CAULIFLOWER	ONION	ZUCCHINI
CELERY		

Vegetables are the main source of carbohydrates on *The Metabolism Solution*. Because most of us cannot spend 20 hours a week exercising to combat insulin resistance and work off the effects of a starchy diet, we need to eat lower amounts of starchy carbohydrates. That's why focusing on veggies is the solution to your weight loss. Vegetables are lower in calories, and you can eat larger portions while still losing weight. By eating more veggies, you minimize your body's demand for insulin and lower your cells' resistance to its effects. These fibrous carbohydrates are not the carbs you need to worry about. They are what I like to call "free food" as most of us don't overeat any type of vegetables; we typically don't eat enough.

DRESS YOUR SALAD LEAN

When I first began trying to lose weight, I switched from hamburgers to salads and couldn't figure out why I wasn't losing weight. I made a common mistake, one you've probably made before too: With all the foods I put in them, my salads were often as calorie-laden as a hamburger. Just because it's called a "salad" doesn't mean it's good for you. Beans, cheese, and egg yolks may be delicious, but they are higher in fat and calories than a burger and fries. Salads need to be delicious, simple, and clean to satisfy while boosting your metabolism. My suggestion: Stick with the lists on these pages.

I avoid bottled dressings by putting vinegar in a spray bottle and misting my salads to coat them evenly and efficiently—no oils. I'm also a big fan of laying HOT fish or chicken on top and letting the juices seep down over my food—then I don't even need dressing. What should you do when you're out at a restaurant? Ask the waiter for vinegar, bring your own dressing, or mix mustard with balsamic vinegar (add 1 Splenda or Truvia if needed) for a delicious dressing or sauce. If you just cannot eat salad or veggies without dressing? That's okay, you'll get there sooner than you think. In the meantime, find your favorite dressing in a fat-free formulation, or the lowest fat and calories you can find. Try cutting it with some vinegar. But let me be honest: It's better to eat salads with a little dressing than to never eat salads at all. If this is what you need to do to get your veggies in, do whatever it takes until you can bear them in a drier state.

There's nothing better than fresh greens with fresh lemon juice and salt and pepper on top. Salad need crunch? Add lightly cooked veggies or cut up carrots to add crunch without loading up on calories. Also, egg whites are a good addition—just leave off the yolk. Hint: Try replacing the oils in your dressings with fat-free chicken broths.

Only the vegetables on my list are metabolic miracles. Eating enough of these vegetables, along with lean proteins, is the solution to boosting your metabolism. If you don't eat enough of them, you slow your metabolism down. Without butter or oil, your body actually uses more calories to digest them than they contain, so you practically end up with a caloric deficit. That's exactly what you want when you're trying to lose weight. All foods have some calories or energy, and all foods require some energy to burn them. It's at this point that the concept of the "negative calorie" comes in. If a food requires more of the body's energy to adequately burn it than the food actually produces, then that food helps create a real thermogenic effect.

As the theory goes, you can eat negative calorie foods to your heart's content and never gain weight. Not only that—you'll lose weight. Vegetables are "careful carbs" that won't affect weight loss unless you don't eat enough of them. If you're not losing weight fast enough, you're probably not eating enough vegetables.

Thermogenic fibrous carbs cause your metabolism to speed up. Combine this with eating clean following *The Metabolism Solution* and your body will incinerate calories at a fat-burning rate. If you've been following the plan exactly, I guarantee it.

You must eat at least five servings (½ cup, unless otherwise noted) a day of these metabolic miracles. Ten servings are even better. Enjoy them steamed, raw, fresh, frozen, or canned (if you must). Just be sure to rinse them thoroughly. I always aim for organic. Please remember: do not add any fats. No butter, no oil. Try sprinkling your vegetables with lemon juice and a pinch of NoSalt and/or pepper (Note: If desired, organic, sea, Himalayan or other salt substitute can be used in all recipes in this book). Or try a dash of balsamic or apple cider vinegar.

Carbohydrates can be quite nutritious, but they do affect blood sugar levels more than

WHAT'S IT GOING TO BE: WINE OR YOUR WAISTLINE?

Alcohol (a carb) and fat loss don't mix. You should refrain from drinking any alcoholic beverages when boosting your metabolism. Your waistline will be glad you did, and you'll feel better. I am always asked how to work alcohol into my diet. The answer is simple: sorry, you can't. Alcohol is second only to dietary fat when it comes to useless calories—not to mention it lowers your resolve, so you end up eating more calories due to blood sugar dips. It doesn't matter if it's clean or organic. Show me a fat stomach and I'll show you a drinker. I recommend not having any until you reach goal weight; and once you arrive, if you insist, have one glass of wine weekly. When alcohol passes the liver, it produces a by-product called acetate which inhibits fat-burning capabilities. The whole purpose of my plan is to rev up your metabolism!

Your body cannot store calories from alcohol for later the way it does with calories from food. When you drink, your metabolism slows down or stops what it is doing (like burning off the calories from your last meal or what you're currently eating) to get rid of the booze. Drinking presses the pause button on your metabolism, pushes away other calories, and says, "Break me down first." The result? What you most recently ate gets stored as fat.

any other food group because we overeat them. Have belly fat? It's a sign you're eating too many carbs. The solution? Cut back—especially on bread and crackers—until you reach your goal weight. And be sure to check labels; carbs sneak in everywhere. Be on guard when buying whey protein shakes or whey protein bars. Many of them contain low-quality carbs—especially sugar—because they are inexpensive to use.

> **WE ONLY NEED ONE-THIRD OF THE CALORIES WE EAT EVERY DAY. REDUCING CARBS IS THE FASTEST WAY TO REDUCE CALORIES.**

Not all carbs are created equal. Vegetable sources are the best and cleanest form of carbohydrates when it comes to boosting your stubborn metabolism. If you are one of the lucky ones who have low body fat and can eat some carbs and keep your weight in check, you can skip this and continue eating carbs the way you always have. But if you want to eat as healthily as possible, choose carbs that are earth-grown such as fresh green veggies for optimal health and nutrients. Yes, carbs can be part of a healthy diet, but if you have ever been overweight and specifically need to lose excess belly and/or thigh fat, this is your body's way of letting you know you need to cut back on carbs; this may or may not include fruits and any carbs found in yogurts or pre-packaged food. It's best and quickest to eliminate carbs while your belly gets lean.

THE NOT-SO-THERMOGENIC CARBS

WHILE THESE FOODS MAY BE CONSIDERED HEALTHY, THEY ALSO SPIKE BLOOD SUGAR LEVELS, WHICH SLOWS THE WEIGHT LOSS PROCESS. THE BOTTOM LINE? THE FEWER CARBS YOU EAT, THE FASTER YOU WILL LOSE WEIGHT. BUT IF YOU NEED TO EAT CARBS, SELECT FROM BELOW.

ALL BRAN (½ CUP)	CORN (½ CUP)	RICE BRAN (½ CUP)
BARLEY (½ CUP)	FIBER ONE CEREAL (½ CUP)	SWEET POTATO (½ CUP)
BEANS – BLACK, FAVA, GARBANZO, KIDNEY, LENTILS, LIMA, NORTHERN, PINTO, RED, SOY, WHITE (2 TBSP.)	OATMEAL (SLOW COOKING, ½ CUP)	WASA LIGHT (1 PIECE)
POPCORN (AIR POPPED, 3 CUPS)	PARSNIPS (½ CUP)	WHOLE GRAIN BREADS (1 OZ.)
	PASTA (½ CUP)	WINTER SQUASH (ALL VARIETIES, ½ CUP)
	BROWN OR WILD RICE (½ CUP)	

Your brain does run on carbs, and it does need glucose for fuel to function properly. But don't worry—your body can and will get the proper fuel from the foods you eat on *The Metabolism Solution*. If you're following this plan, eating an apple every day, and loading up on veggies, you'll be lean in no time, and your body will get the carbohydrates it needs to function and fuel your body and brain. When you overeat carbohydrates—like when you eat out and have more than half a cup of pasta, a piece of bread, and dessert—your body pumps out insulin, a hormone to keep your blood sugar within a certain range (otherwise your brain would go haywire). Insulin is also a powerful fat-storage hormone, so your body stores the excess sugar as fat. This is especially true under stressful conditions when your cortisol levels are high. Go ahead; take a look at your middle. Are you storing excess fat in this area?

When you overload on carbs, it doesn't matter what you're eating, even if it's the gourmet "health" carb of the month like quinoa. Once you replace your current diet with lean proteins and vegetables, your stomach will disappear quickly, and you'll lose weight easily.

What separates the good carbs from the bad? When it comes to boosting your metabolism, only carbohydrates that come from a high-fiber vegetable source fit the bill. We only need one-third of the calories we eat every day, and reducing the bad carbs is the fastest way to reduce calories. I'm sorry to be the bearer of this news (don't shoot the messenger), but as America gets fatter and unhealthier due to the rise in blood-sugar levels, I have to tell you the truth: You need to cut down on non-vegetable carbs. You especially need to cut down on carbohydrates as you age and your activity decreases. Your body doesn't process carbs the same at 45 as it did at 25. So skip the carbs. If you really must eat carbs, be sure to always pair them with a lean protein to slow the carbs from being broken down into sugars.

A LITTLE FAT IS ALL YOU NEED

Yes, you do need fat, but not as much as you may think. When it comes to losing weight, we need less because we already have enough fat stored. A woman needs about 15 grams of fat a day, while men and teenagers both get 20 grams. This is where most people get stymied in their weight loss because they are unaware of where fats lurk in food. And just because a fat is good for you, doesn't mean you can eat more of it. Fats, saturated and not, are still bad for weight loss. Fat portions may be extremely small, but they have an extremely high calorie count. You need less fat in your daily diet than you think, and you are probably already eating more of it than you realize.

Fats are a very important nutrient group. You must take in adequate essential fats or your body will not burn fat. Essential fats are very important for skin, hair, and nails and many other bodily functions. Fat adds taste and usually makes you feel full and satiated. I say "usually" because most of us who are or have been overweight lack an "I'm full" switch and overeat on fat too. Diets high in fat slow down your metabolism. Why would your body burn off stored fat if you are still eating enough? Your body will let go of fat when you stop overeating it.

For the fastest weight loss, I strongly suggest that you supplement with an omega-3 capsule to meet your fat needs. While an omega-3 capsule meets your dietary fat needs, I know it probably won't meet your taste needs.

I live in the real world, too. It's super important to avoid the bad fats or any fat that you can't measure or control the amount you eat. Consume too much, even if it's a good fat, and you won't lose weight. Just about all processed foods are high in bad fats and should be avoided for fast weight loss.

Bad fats contain larger amounts of partially saturated, saturated, and trans-fatty acids. These fats are common in processed foods such as fried foods, beef, pork, lamb, cheese, cream, butter, milk, and nut butters (both processed and unprocessed). The foods that contain fat (including "health" foods) may shock you. Maybe you've been eating them all along and wondering why you are not losing weight.

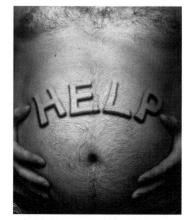

The list of healthy fats includes avocados, nuts, and oils—both in supplements as well as cooking oils. Use them sparingly. Don't fall into the temptation of thinking that just because they appear on a "healthy" list that you can't overdo the amount you consume, because you certainly can. Don't be one of those who eat an entire half gallon of low or reduced fat ice cream just because it's "healthy." This is simply a marketing ploy and will derail your weight loss efforts in a hurry. Always read labels and check for the number of fat grams.

Don't let belly fat hold you hostage

Nevertheless, the right amount of good fat is a great thing for your metabolism. Good fats contain the essential fatty acids (like fish oil) that your body cannot make on its own and play a vital role in virtually every bodily function. You want these oils to be as pure as possible, and you must measure them carefully. More is definitely not better. You can periodically include oils such as olive oil or a very small handful of nuts (one ounce in a serving—be sure to measure) once daily. This is where a small slice of avocado works if you crave it.

I recommend only one tablespoon per day earlier in the day so your body has time to use it rather than store it when your metabolism naturally slows down at night to prepare for sleep. Do not consume any other fats. No butter, cream, whole milk, or red meat. They are non-essential. Not needed. They will only do your body harm and stop the whole fat loss process. Be sure to monitor portion size (measure it out) because even essential fats can and will be stored. For fast fat loss, enhance your diet with a quality omega-3 supplement to give your body what it needs.

FRUIT: TOO MUCH OF A GOOD THING?

Fruit is one of the easiest snacks and desserts to transport. And while delicious, it is critical that you understand that it's not "free" like vegetables under *The Metabolism Solution*. Fruit contains sugar, and even though it's natural, it still has an effect on blood sugar. When it comes to boosting metabolism, sugar is sugar. It doesn't really matter where it comes from. Fruit does contain fiber that helps slow absorption, keeps you feeling full, and contains nutrients your body needs; nevertheless, vegetables beat fruit for fat loss.

Fruit converts to sugar very quickly during digestion. This not only stops the fat-burning process but helps your body store fat. Just as with fats, try to consume fruit early in the day (never past three in the afternoon). Grapefruits and apples (especially Granny Smith) are fairly low on the glycemic index. Also, berries (strawberries, blueberries, blackberries, and raspberries) are low in sugar and higher in fiber than other fruits. Limit melons, mangoes, and pineapples. These are very high in sugar and are

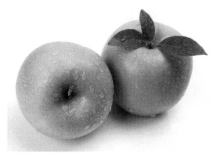

probably best avoided if you cannot manage portion control. However, it is always better to overeat on fruit than cookies, brownies, potato chips, or other junk food. Just keep this information in mind while trying to lose body fat.

Limit your fruit to one to two servings a day. I always suggest a green apple for a 3:00 p.m. snack. Be sure to measure the amount you eat. Too much, even of a good thing, may be the culprit in your inability to lose weight. Any diabetic will tell you how their blood sugar rises after eating fruit.

Try a green apple for a 3:00p.m. snack

YOUR SUGAR FIX: LOW-SUGAR FRUITS

Fruit, high in enzymes and minerals, is nature's cleanser.
Enjoy two fruits per day maximum.
One portion is one half cup unless otherwise noted.
Fresh or frozen (without added sugar) is fine.
Always choose organic.

APPLES, GRANNY SMITH ARE BEST (1 SMALL)	**ALL MELONS (½ CUP)**
BLUEBERRIES (1 CUP)	**GRAPEFRUIT (½ SMALL OR ½ CUP)**
BLACKBERRIES (1 CUP)	**KIWI (1 SMALL)**
	CHERRIES (10 LARGE)

SUGAR SUBSTITUTES: THE FACTS WITHOUT ALL THE HYPE

Did you know that the average American consumes three pounds of sugar a week? Blame sugar for obesity, hypertension, fatigue, high blood pressure, headaches, and the metabolic meltdown we are facing in this country. Sugar is as addictive as cocaine. If you're trying to lose weight, shed belly fat, or just eat healthier, you know that reducing the amount of sugar you eat is one of the most important steps in the process. So when you want something sweet, where do you turn? Artificial sweeteners or other sugar substitutes. There are pros and cons when it comes to using sugar substitutes, both artificial and natural-based. I'm not a proponent of using them, but I'm also not against using them in moderation. I find it helpful to have a diet soda instead of a bag of "gourmet health chips"—I feel a lot less guilt. Some top brands you can find today include:

- AGAVE NECTAR comes from the agave plant and is sweeter than honey. Use carefully as it is very high in fructose, which can super-spike blood sugar.
- EQUAL was the first aspartame sweetener sold to the public, hitting the market in 1981. Aspartame safety has been debated over the years, but research studies deem it fine for use.
- NUTRASWEET is another aspartame sweetener.
- SPLENDA is a sucralose-based sweetener that hit the U.S. market in 1999. It is the leading brand in the United States with 60 percent of the sugar-substitute market. Sucralose does not affect blood sugar, and it is what I use.
- SWEET 'N LOW is a saccharin-based sugar substitute. Saccharin has fallen out of favor after some research from the 1970s linked it to cancer in rats. According to the National Cancer Institute, however, subsequent studies have not proven a connection.
- TRUVIA is a stevia-based sweetener. Stevia is a South American plant and was approved as a general-use sugar substitute in 2008. In studies, it did not affect blood sugar of those with Type 2 Diabetes or healthy people. Truvia is now the number two sugar substitute in the United States after Splenda.

DAIRY, THE WANNABE PROTEIN

Milk-based protein is an inferior source of protein and does not possess the same metabolic-boosting properties as whey whey protein. Milk is high in sugar and lactose, which is of course detrimental for weight loss and can cause digestive issues. The calcium content is often minimal. Most commercially bought shakes and all protein bars are made from milk-based proteins—that's how they keep their

prices so low. Regardless of what the label or commercial tells you, dairy will not keep you tight and lean. I have met and helped so many people who are doing almost everything right, except for the fact that they eat dairy daily and cannot understand why they are not losing weight. The low-fat yogurt you favor may have protein; but it's not whey, and it's usually full of sugar, too. Whey-based protein is protein derived from the watery portion of milk when making

NONDAIRY CREAMERS (low-fat and nonfat alike) are your enemies when it comes to boosting your metabolism. Don't let that "little bit" fool you. Drink your coffee black or add a little bit of your protein shake and watch the pounds fall off quickly.

cheese, thus, you get the nutritional benefits of dairy without the fat. My clients who are fitness models and bodybuilders will not eat any dairy at all for a year before a show to really lean out. Foregoing dairy causes their skin to become thin and tight, and this allows you to see the fine-tuned musculature on their bodies.

That being said, this is the real world, and you do need variety. I like to think of this food group, dairy, as dessert. I don't count it toward my total of protein for the day but eat it as a dessert in addition to my total. I have a small child's cone of frozen yogurt every day as a treat (I told you I wasn't perfect). This trick has kept me on track for over 20 years because I know I can have it daily, and it satisfies me because dairy takes a long time to digest and keeps me feeling full. Keep in mind, I've already had a quality whey protein shake to boost my metabolism—this is simply dessert. If I am having a slow day and not eating enough protein, I will add one scoop of the shake to my yogurt to guarantee that my very slow metabolism gets what it needs.

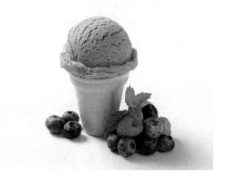

The dairy listed below should be used sparingly, if at all, until you reach your goal weight. At that time you can add a little bit back into your diet. I recommend adding one very small serving at a time and keeping a close eye on the scale to see if you gain weight—if you do, you'll know why. Note that soy and rice milk are simply not good sources of protein because they are missing amino acids and are not a complete protein like whey.

Dairy Is for Cows and Kids—Not Fat Loss

NONFAT CHEESE, PREFERABLY VEGETA-
BLE-BASED (1 OZ.)

NONFAT COTTAGE CHEESE (½ CUP)

NONFAT RICOTTA CHEESE (½ CUP)

NONFAT/NO-SUGAR YOGURT (FRESH OR FRO-
ZEN, ½ CUP)

SKIM MILK (1 CUP)

COCONUT MILK (½ CUP)

RICE MILK/PLAIN UNSWEETENED (½ CUP)

SOY MILK/PLAIN UNSWEETENED (½ CUP)

THERMOGENIC CONDIMENTS AND SEASONINGS

No fats, no sauces, no cheeses. I can hear the groans. There are tasty replacements for these weight-gain-inducing extras that can imbue your lean proteins and vegetables with mouth-watering fla-

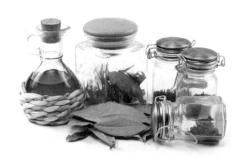

vors. It's true; when you cut the fat, you tend to cut a lot of flavor too. Learning how to season your food without relying on fats is easy. You can add a lot of flavor without the calories. Every lean kitchen must have low-calorie, low-fat, and low-sodium seasoning staples.

Try to avoid soy, a metabolism-slowing ingredient that is in just about every marinade on the store shelf. When buying broth, look for organic, gluten-free, and those that contain as little sodium as possible. It can often be substituted in place of an oil, in a homemade salad dress-

ing for example. Aromatics such as scallions, onions, ginger, garlic, and lemongrass all fall into this group. The name tells you everything you need to know, and they add that wow factor to your foods by making them smell good and taste amazing.

Many spices not only add flavor but have health benefits as well. Cinnamon may help regulate blood sugar; turmeric can help you burn fat since its main component is curcumin, which is a diarylhepta-noid or secondary metabolite. And don't forget about metabolism-boosting cayenne. Its main ingredient, capsaicin, suppresses your appetite and helps burn fat.

**Statistics Show That You Are Guaranteed to Have a Weight Problem
If You Eat Out More Than One Meal a Week. How You Can Avoid the Weight Gain?**

1. BOOST YOUR METABOLISM. Drink a protein shake for two meals before and after you eat out to offset the calories, balance your sugar levels, and boost your metabolism.
2. BLOCK CARBS AND KILL CRAVINGS. Studies have shown that white kidney bean extract blocks up to 65 percent of unwanted carbs from being broken down and stored as fat.
3. DRINK AT LEAST TWO LARGE GLASSES OF WATER BEFORE YOUR MEAL. Do not indulge in alcohol. Try a cup of hot tea to fill you up. At a party? Have some diet ginger ale in a champagne glass.
4. KNOW BEFORE YOU GO. Check the menu online or call ahead before you select a restaurant to avoid getting stuck with fat-inducing choices. Choose what you'll eat before you get there. Many restaurants also offer a "light" menu. Select from it, and you can save 800 or more calories.
5. EAT YOUR VEGETABLES. All 10 servings. Focus on eating steamed veggies with sauces on the side—and ask that they be prepared without butter.
6. SLIM DOWN YOUR SALAD AND EAT AS MUCH AS YOU CAN. You'll be fuller by the time the entrée is served, and that will help you avoid temptation. To keep your salad lean, say yes to vegetables but "no" to avocado, cheese, beans, croutons, raisins (all dried fruit), bacon, yolks, and nuts. Pick a vinaigrette over a creamy dressing option. Or try my secret dressing: mustard mixed with vinegar. Top it all off with shrimp or salmon. You can save up to 800 calories.
7. SHARING IS CARING. Split an entree with your dinner companion or ask the waiter to wrap up half of your entree to take home for tomorrow. You'll save both calories and money.
8. FILL UP WITH BROTH. Broth-based soups like chicken noodle (without the noodles), minestrone, garden vegetable, and miso save hundreds of calories and keep you full and satisfied.

TRY THESE THIRST-QUENCHING, DELICIOUS, AND HYDRATING TRICKS TO ENCOURAGE YOU TO DRINK MORE WATER

1. Water with lemon or lime. It's light and fresh.
2. Add cinnamon to create a slimming water.
3. Try cucumbers and ginger for an irresistible, fresh, clean treat.
4. Water with floating fruit. Using whatever fruit you have on hand— citrus, berries, apples, nectarines, you name it—slice and add to a large pitcher of water. Kids will love the juicy fruit when the water is gone.
5. Skinny hot chocolate. This is my personal favorite. Mix 1 scoop of chocolate protein powder with water. Warm it up (do not boil) for a skinny hot chocolate treat.
6. Coffee and tea—hot or cold. Just hold the sugar and dairy. Diet bottled teas are okay every now and then.
7. Zero-calorie flavored waters. Packets or already bottled.
8. Sparkling waters (carbonated waters as well as mineral waters) such as Perrier and Pellegrino, seltzers (flavored and plain), and club soda. Try a splash (and I mean a quick splash—not a glass) of juice in your seltzer as you wean yourself from sugary drinks.
9. Make flavored ice cubes using any of the above calorie-free drinks and add them to your water.

DRINK MORE WATER, BOOST YOUR METABOLISM THREE PERCENT

Did you know that, 9 times out of 10 when you think your body is sending you hunger signals, they're really thirst signals? Dehydration can slow your metabolism by three percent. Getting enough water helps your body cleanse itself and flush out waste. It is imperative to drink half your body weight in ounces of water daily. That may sound like a lot, but it's not that bad. Weigh 150 pounds? That's 75 ounces of water, which is about 4½ standard-sized (16.9 oz.) water bottles a day.

For some of you that may be easy; for me—not so much. I need a little motivation when it comes to drinking water. I love pure, ice-cold water when I'm working out, but at other times, I add calorie-free, fat-free flavor to entice my taste buds to reach for a bottle of water. I also leave visual cues to get myself to drink. An eye-catching pitcher of water left on a counter alongside a pretty glass reminds me to stop and drink every time I walk by. I love to add cucumber slices with ginger or lemon slices to my pitcher. I've even been known to add the occasional melon ball or two.

I've been asked many times about the sugar-free packets made to add to bottled water. While not ideal, they work in a pinch. I keep the little packets of Crystal Light Peach Iced Tea and Lemonade in my purse and at my home to add to water when I'm desperate and haven't been drinking like I should.

These packets help promote water drinking, and drinking water always keeps you from overeating. Drink at least two large glasses of water before

THERMOGENIC EATING FOR RADICAL WEIGHT LOSS

your meals, and you can lose an average of 16 pounds in 3 months.

Remember: When you think you're hungry, you are many times actually thirsty. Before you reach for something to chew, try a drink first. These are my favorite calorie-free beverages (and they count toward your ounces of water) that keep me—and will keep you—satisfied and feeling full. They hit the spot without adding any extra calories. Try them cold or hot; just don't add a drop of dairy.

THE LEGAL SNACK ATTACK

It happens to me, too. I have those moments where I just can't help myself. Sometimes, you just need to eat, even when you know you shouldn't. There are foods that are helpful to have on hand for such binge moments. But when it comes to foods you can or cannot eat, remember: when in doubt, don't! Stay away from foods you might binge on; it will slow your weight loss, you'll have too much guilt, and it won't be worth it. Before you start that binge, ask yourself what you're really feeling.

If snack you must, choose foods with the lowest caloric content such as those on the list below. I'll be honest. When I'm truly craving, it's for something I want tzo nosh a lot of, not simply "snack." That's why this list is made up of high-volume, low-calorie foods that won't have you going over your calorie budget when you have more than just one. Always make sure that you have eaten 10 servings of vegetables. If you're still looking for more food, you might be wanting more because you didn't eat your 10 vegetables.

WAIT, DON'T REACH FOR THAT DOUGHNUT!

Bumps on the road to weight loss show up in a food journal. A journal helps diagnose the behavior behind your overeating. Once you address the behavior, the problem (overeating) takes care of itself. Here are some tips on avoiding these obstacles.

- **Bored?** Tackle an item on your to-do list.
- **Lonely?** Call a friend.
- **Poor planning?** Make a plan or plan to fail.
- **Angry?** Exercise instead.
- **Craving crunch?** Popcorn or veggies satisfy that need.
- **Craving comfort?** Make a cup of Skinny Hot Chocolate.
- **Tired?** Take a nap or go to bed earlier.
- **At a restaurant?** Plan what you will eat ahead of time.
- **Hungry outside meal times?** Drink a glass of water and journal instead.

- Air-Popped Popcorn, 3 cups (60 calories)
- Clear Broth Soup
- Fudgesicles (25 to 40 calories)
- Garden Salad
- Green Apple, 1 small
- Sugarless gum
- Sugar-Free Candy, 2 pieces
- Sugar-Free Gelatin
- Sugar-Free Popsicles (15 to 25 calories)
- Tomato Juice
- Tootsie Roll Pop (25 calories)

WHO SAID CHEATERS NEVER LOSE?

If you are stuck on a weight loss plateau or you need to lose those last stubborn five to ten pounds, cheating the right way on your diet may be exactly what your body needs. Now don't get too excited; this is not a license to eat whatever and how much you want. Overindulging without forethought can require up to a solid week of clean eating to get back on track.

The secret to cheating without gaining an ounce is to prepare your metabolism ahead of time—boost your metabolism before you indulge so that when you do cheat, your body is ready to torch those calories instead of storing them. Boosting your metabolism and then cheating sends your metabolic fire into fireball mode. The metabolic bonfire will power you through that plateau and blast off that extra five to ten pounds.

Don't worry if you fall off the wagon. You are human, and it's expected because no one is perfect. Just know that 80% is as good as you'll get, even when it comes to staying on your weight loss plan. Let it go and get right back on. Fix a binge in one day by going back to the 48-Hour Metabolic Boosting Cleanse (see page 119). It can boost your metabolism and fix your worst eating day.

RULES AND NUMBERS FOR WEIGHT LOSS

The most effective way to lose weight is to follow a strict, structured plan. It works faster and is 10 times more effective than putting a plan together yourself. Whether following a plan or trying to create your own, you must stick with foods that boost your metabolism. Math is important to weight loss success. Never forget this formula for your daily calorie requirement. These numbers are critical when trying to lose weight.

YOUR GOAL WEIGHT X 10 = TOTAL CALORIES FOR THE DAY

So if you are reaching for 120 pounds, you need to consume 1,200 calories maximum per day to hit that goal. *The Metabolism Solution* has this already taken care of, but if you decide to try the do-it-your-self approach, here's what you need to know:

1. **Start your day with whey to boost your metabolism by 25 percent.** Within one hour of waking, drink a whey-based protein shake.
2. **Limit fat.** Keep your daily fat intake to 15 grams max for women and 20 grams max for men and teens. Choose only essential fats.
3. **Be careful with carbs.** Consume non-vegetable carbohydrates (if you insist on eating them) before 3:00 p.m. If you're losing too slowly, drop carbs completely (vegetables do not count). Keep your non-vegetable carbs to less than 75 grams per day.
4. **Power your metabolism with protein.** Consume 25 grams of lean protein (see list) per meal.
5. **Read labels to be lean.** Check calorie counts. Weigh or measure everything you eat, then calculate your calorie intake using a calorie book or website. This one simple step can make or break your weight loss.
6. **Water for weight loss.** Drink half your body weight in ounces of water daily. That's typi-cally 8 to 10 8-oz. glasses a day—minimum.
7. **Snack slim.** Keep snacks at 100 calories or less. Better yet, snack on veggies or fruit.
8. **Timing is everything.** Keep a minimum of three hours between meals. If you eat in be-tween, your body cannot digest the food and will store it as fat. This could also cause insulin to rise and slow down all the metabolic boosting you've been working so hard to create.
9. **Food is only half your day.** Eat all your meals in a 12-hour window (7:00 a.m. to 7:00 p.m., for example).
10. **Get HUNGRY!** Hunger is a good sign. It means your body is about to burn fat. The feeling will dissipate. You don't need to instantly gratify every food craving. Find another way to entertain yourself—change a thought and move muscle, anything BUT succumb to eating again. You will not be literally starving. It was a pivotal moment for me when I learned it was okay to be hungry. Hunger is a sign your body is about to start burning fat. Don't let it scare you.

IF YOU BITE IT, WRITE IT!

In the last 25 years, I have learned a lot about how food journals can be helpful. But I've also learned that most people don't use them enough and aren't always totally honest when they do. Honest food journals work—studies show that people who journal exactly what they ate lost more weight and kept it off. What I find helps the most is

> **IF YOU BITE IT, WRITE IT! EVERY MORSEL OF IT. THE GOOD DAYS AREN'T NECES-SARY; LOG THE REALLY BAD ONES FOR BEST INSIGHT.**

logging your bad days for true insight on you and food.

If you bite, chew, sip, or chug it, write it down. What you eat in private shows up on the scale (or your body), so be honest with yourself. Be sure to add what you put on your food or in your coffee, as it's these small things that often add up and cause us to gain weight in the first place. List how much of each food you eat, the time of day, and how you felt when you ate it. Did you eat standing up in front of the refrigerator? Or were you sitting down, eating slowly in a relaxed state? All of this matters. Rate your hunger on a scale from 1 to 5 with 5 being the most hungry (real hunger, not head hunger) and record that too. After all, most of the eating we do isn't real hunger at all but rather stress showing up in our food consumption habits.

Metabolic Boosting Food Journal

Use this checklist to help you stay on track every day. Be sure to write down everything you eat each day and mark off the corresponding box. The number of boxes shown for each food group is the number of servings to be eaten each day. If you notice several blank boxes, focus on eating foods from the missing groups to BOOST your metabolism. Don't forget to check off your exercise and supplement boxes.

	SUNDAY	MONDAY	TUESDAY	WEDNESDAY	THURSDAY	FRIDAY	SATURDAY	SUNDAY
Water	○○○○○ ○○○○○	○○○○○ ○○○○○	○○○○○ ○○○○○	○○○○○ ○○○○○	○○○○○ ○○○○○	○○○○○ ○○○○○	○○○○○ ○○○○○	○○○○○ ○○○○○
Protein Shake/ Bar	○○	○○	○○	○○	○○	○○	○○	○○
Vegetables	○○○○○ ○○○○○	○○○○○ ○○○○○	○○○○○ ○○○○○	○○○○○ ○○○○○	○○○○○ ○○○○○	○○○○○ ○○○○○	○○○○○ ○○○○○	○○○○○ ○○○○○
Fish/Protein	○	○	○	○	○	○	○	○
Fruit	○	○	○	○	○	○	○	○
Snack	○	○	○	○	○	○	○	○
Supplements/AM	○	○	○	○	○	○	○	○
Supplements/PM	○	○	○	○	○	○	○	○
Sleep (list hours)								WORSHIP!
Pray/Meditate (check)								
Cardio (list length)								
Metabolic Workouts #								
Body Weight/BMI								

Lean Proteins	Veggies	Low Sugar Fruits	Calorie Free Beverages	Snacks	Supplements For Fat Loss
Protein Shake	All Lettuce - 3 cups	Apple - 1 small	Water	Protein Bar	Protein Shake
Egg Whites - 3	Spinach - 1/2 cup	Blueberries - 1/2 cup	Green Tea	Cut-up Veggies	Protein Bar
All Fish - 4oz.	All Green Veggies - 1/2 cup	Raspberries - 1/2 cup	Black Coffee	Protein Shake	(watch sugar/carb content)
Turkey - 3oz.	Cabbage - 1 cup	Grapefruit - 1/2 cup	Calorie-Free Seltzer	Sugar-free, Fat-free Jell-O	Omega-3, Raspberry Ketone
Chicken Breast - 3oz.	Broccoli - 1/2 cup			15-calorie Popsicles/Fudgesicles	Green Tea
Protein Bar	String Beans - 1 cup			3 Cups Air-popped Popcorn	Cocoa Bean Powder
	Brussel Sprouts - 1 cup			Pudding Cups < 100 calories	Forskolin, Banaba Leaf
	Zucchini - 1 cup			100 Calorie Popcorn	Gugglesterones
	Yellow Squash - 1 cup	Visit **LynFit.com** today for more metabolic boosting		(6) Almonds < 100 calories	White Kidney Bean Extract
	Peas - 1/2 cup	information		Yogurt < 100 calories	Melatonin (bedtime)
				Tic Tacs	Vitamin D

Researchers from the Fred Hutchinson Cancer Research Center found that dieters who kept food journals lost six pounds more than those who didn't journal. And that's not even the best part. Food journals have proven to be more helpful than simply serving as a list to keep track of what you eat. They keep you accountable for what you put in your mouth and tip you off to your emotional triggers that cause overeating. Food journaling reveals if you skip meals, eat out often, or neglect meal planning—behaviors which can lead to overeating. Once revealed, these behaviors can be addressed. It's also critical to journal where you are while you are eating and your feelings at that moment. Were you out with friends? Alone? Upset over a disagreement with a loved one? These kinds of situations very much affect weight loss if you respond to them with food.

After much research, I use the food journal shown in this chapter with my clients. (You can also download it from my website at www.lynfit.com.) It allows you to check off supplements as well. While it is extremely helpful and useful for keeping track of what you eat, it only works if you're honest. That's why I'm especially asking you to track your bad days. From those days in particular, you can learn what needs to be changed about how you eat. Remember, what you eat accounts for 80 percent, if not more, of your battle to lose weight. Take a moment and enter your food intake in a journal. Be sure to write what you were feeling before you ate as well as what you craved. That will help you troubleshoot in the future. Journals aren't about creating more work; they are a way to track so you can look back and determine where you went off course.

THE DIET DIAGNOSER

Use the following questions to determine what you are doing right and wrong concerning your daily food intake. This is the fastest way to figure out where you are "off" so that you know exactly what you need to do to lose weight today.

1. Did you drink a whey protein shake at least once without adding fruit or dairy?
2. Did you eat vegetables? Were they greens or high-sugar types like carrots and tomatoes?
3. Did you drink 10 glasses of water?
4. Did you eat carbs? (Be on carb alert. They show up everywhere; check all your labels.)
5. Did you "slip up" on any of the following diet destroyers:
   - Cheese
   - Milk (Soy or Other)
   - Oils
   - Nuts
   - Red Meat
   - Alcohol
   - Candy or Cookies
   - Pasta
   - Bread
   - Excess Fruit
6. Have you weighed and measured everything?
7. Did you forget to take the supplements your metabolism requires for weight loss?
8. Did you walk every day for 45 minutes to an hour?
9. Did you do the Metabolic Boosting Workouts? They're "medicine" for your metabolism.
10. Are you worried that you won't lose weight and, as a result, so stressed that it's affecting your weight loss?

I assure you—*The Metabolism Solution* works every time when you follow it. Everyone loses weight. No one fails. So if the scale is stuck, it's time to slip out of diet denial and keep reassessing what you're eating until you find the weight gain culprit. It took me years to figure this out. The truth was that I didn't want to admit or accept that the "little bit" of raisins or milk or my once-a-week breakfast of oatmeal could do so much harm. Once I decided to stop eating these foods, the scale dropped right away. You have to challenge yourself—step out of your comfort zone—if you are serious about boosting your metabolism to lose weight faster.

CLEANSE, BOOST, REPEAT

The goal is to not only eat healthy (as eating from the lists of foods on the preceding pages will have you do) but also lose weight. So, to jumpstart your metabolism, you need to reboot it. That's where my cleanse comes in. The average cleanse—and there are many to choose from on the market—purports to detoxify and heal your body, mostly by eliminating waste and not necessarily nourishing the rest of you. Detoxifying is important because it helps make it easier for your body to burn calories, but detoxifying the wrong way will damage your metabolism and make weight loss even more difficult.

Juicing has been popular for years now, but it's not a good plan to follow for weight loss. While you might lose a pound or two because you're only drinking and not eating for a day or more, juiced vegetables and fruits will jackhammer your blood sugar through the roof. And are you going to be able to keep that pound off and build on it? You can juice to your heart's content, but you will not find a faster or better way to boost your metabolism than the Metabolic Boosting Cleanse. The best part? You get to eat, not just drink. Eating and chewing your food (and especially your vegetables) is always best because then you're burning calories during digestion. Juicing breaks down food into such small particles that they are digested very quickly, not requiring as many calories for the process. And when food digests so quickly, your blood sugar spikes and causes your body to store fat, specifically around the midsection, hips, and thighs. I call this "the insulin band," and if you wear such a band, it's proof positive that you're eating too many of the wrong carbohydrates and sugars.

> **HOW DO YOU KNOW if you need to cleanse? Here are the telltale signs that your body is begging for one:**
> - Cravings
> - Bloating, feeling heavy, constipation
> - Hard time losing weight
> - Depression, moodiness
> - Tired, lacking energy
> - Muscle aches and pains
> - Sleep problems
> - Skin eruptions/eczema
> - Sick, frequent colds/headaches
> - Sinus and allergy problems

The Metabolic-Boosting Cleanse

The very best way to start off your journey on *The Metabolism Solution* program is with my jumpstart cleanse. You will detoxify your body in a healthy way while rebooting your whole system. Trust me, it works! The sample day below is a guide to experiencing the best possible Metabolic-Boosting Cleanse. Your high-quality whey protein shakes will start your metabolism off like a furnace each day, and everything you consume during your cleanse works to get your metabolism into tip-top, calorie-incinerating shape.

BREAKFAST
- High-quality whey protein shake
- Multivitamin to provide nutrients and energy
- Green tea as desired throughout day

LUNCH
- Complete whey protein shake

MIDDAY
- 1 omega-3 capsule to curb cravings

DINNER
- Green vegetables (5 ½-cup servings) and white fish (4 oz.)
- 2 raspberry keytone supplements

BEDTIME
- Melatonin to provide restful and revitalizing sleep

It's called a "cleanse" because it alkalinizes your body, returning it to its proper pH levels (sweets, meats, and processed foods create acidity), detoxifies, and reboots your metabolism; but it is so much more. Cleansing is the important first step on the road to weight loss following *The Metabolism Solution*. The Metabolic Boosting Cleanse is the fastest, safest cleanse on the market, and the best part is that it's so safe you can repeat it as often as needed. In fact, some of my clients feel so much better on it that they follow the cleanse and live on it two to three days a week as a way to control their weight, gain health and feel better. Can you say that about any other cleanse?

You start the cleanse the way I recommend you start every morning—with a high-quality whey protein shake, which feeds the muscle and starves the fat. You won't find high-quality whey protein in a juice cleanse. Lunch is the same. For a change of pace, check out my shake recipes; and for a truly met-

THE LEAN GREEN CLEANSING MACHINE

Cleansing is the best way to jumpstart your fat loss when you do it right. Try this reenergizing and detoxifying shake to put you on the weight loss path. Scared you won't like the veggies in it? Start slow and try one new veggie each day. Most people love kale, cucumber, and spinach because they taste so mild.

- **1 cup water or black coffee (coffee is loaded with antioxidants)**
- **2 scoops of your favorite high-quality whey protein shake**
- **1 large cucumber**
- **1 fistful of kale**
- **1 stalk of celery**
- **1 large broccoli floret with stem**
- **½ peeled lemon**

Wash and prep ingredients. Add to blender and blend away. Makes two servings—so drink half for breakfast and save the rest for lunch!

abolic-revving alternative, add some greens. You read that right. Who knew that kale, cucumber, and celery could taste so cool and refreshing in a vanilla whey protein shake?

There's no snacking between meals, but you can fill up on green tea, which is full of antioxidants. Give your body time to digest what you consume, wait at least three hours between meals, and let yourself feel hungry—that's a sign your body is burning fat. Dinner consists of vegetables and a lean, clean, white protein like fish. White fish is preferred over salmon, chicken, and turkey because it is less fatty. Think green and white when it comes to food: green for vegetables and white for fish. These are the foods that meet your body's needs and boost your metabolism. And don't forget to drink plenty of water—10 8-oz. glasses a day (green tea counts toward the requirement).

Supplements are key to the entire process. While on a cleanse, they are best way to ensure your body gets the nutrients needed while your food intake is low. A multivitamin in the morning, an Omega-3 capsule at 3:00 p.m., two raspberry ketone supplements with dinner, and a melatonin just before bedtime will provide even more "punch" to your cleanse. During sleep is when true detoxing takes place, so it's best to sleep seven to eight hours per night.

Once you've started the reboot of your metabolism with the cleanse, you have completed the first steps to weight loss and can add some additional foods to your dinner and later your lunch (stick with those on the lists). Throw out all of the junk food you have lying around. Prepare by going shopping and buying only what you need. Bring the food lists with you. If you need to eat out, call the restaurant ahead of time and ask them to prepare your fish and green salad without dressing, croutons, or cheese. Broil your fish with lemon juice instead of butter, oil, or any extra NoSalt. Then sit down and write out your meals—and be exact. Write down what you will eat and when. Keep in mind that it's best to eat between the hours of 7:00 a.m. and 7:00 p.m., but definitely no later than 8:00 p.m.

After cleansing for two or three days, you can vary your dinner once in a while by having 3 ounces of chicken and at 3:00 p.m. adding a snack of a green apple or other legal snack. If you stick to this Metabolic-Boosting Meal Plan, you can lose up to one pound per day. The key words here are, "If you stick to it."

What about constipation? Staying regular is crucial during this time, but you don't want to spend your day in the bathroom either, which is how some cleanses operate. If you're eating enough veggies and drinking enough water, you will be regular. Aim for 10 veggie servings per day minimum.

One final thing to consider while losing weight using *The Metabolism Solution* is the use of over-the-counter medication, much of which is metabolism-deadening—particularly antihistamines. If you can, check with your doctor and consider not taking them. You may very well find you can do without them once you detoxify and begin eating clean.

> THE GREATER THE VARIETY OF FOODS IN YOUR HOUSE, THE MORE LIKELY YOU ARE TO HAVE A WEIGHT PROBLEM.
> KEEP IT SIMPLE.

The average weight-loss program is full of don'ts. Don't eat this and don't eat that. Don't ever eat entire categories of food. I want you to enjoy food. Nevertheless, if you want to lose weight and keep it off, you have to make changes to your diet to see changes in your body. I still live to eat, and what I've come to realize is that successful weight loss lies in replacing favorite foods with lighter, leaner versions and having a high-quality whey protein shake. Use the foods found on the preceding lists to create a meal plan that suits you best. Remember the following "musts."

1. Drink a high-quality whey protein shake for breakfast every day.
2. Drink at least 10 cups of water a day.
3. Eat 10 vegetable servings per day.
4. Keep a three-hour minimum and four-hour maximum between meals to keep your blood sugar levels balanced.
5. Eat right at night by choosing a four-ounce serving of lean protein and at least five vegetables for dinner.

For leanest results, do not drink acoloholic beverages or any juice. Try to fit your meals into a 12-hour window (breakfast at 7:00 a.m., lunch at 1:00 p.m., and dinner at 7:00 p.m. Do not eat after 8:00 p.m.).

Remember, it's always better to eat frozen vegetables than none at all and adding a lean protein to the veggies makes it a complete meal. When you are feeding a whole family dinner, I rely on the recipes in chapter seven. With these, it's easy to design a seven-day dinner plan that works for everyone; I base my family's meals on it.

There's something to be said for sticking to the same daily meals. Dieters who eat the same foods daily not only lose more weight faster but also keep it off longer. You can take the guesswork out of meal planning by creating a family meal calendar and sticking with it. Your life will be easier, and you'll live leaner.

METABOLIC-BOOSTING MEAL PLAN

Keep in mind that exercise is important in so many ways, but it's truly what and how much you eat that really determines your weight loss. This is the base plan that you can stick with for the rest of your life. No one is perfect; you will sneak in foods and entire meals that you shouldn't, but as long as you get back on the plan, you'll get back to losing weight and keeping it off.

Starting your day with a high-quality whey protein shake makes all the difference. This one drink revs up your metabolism for the rest of the day. If you just replace your usual breakfast with a whey protein shake, you'll see a difference. But if you follow *The Metabolism Solution*, you'll see real change.

Once the weight begins to come off, you can replace your lunch-time shake with vegetables and a lean protein. You'll find plenty of satisfying and filling foods to choose from within these pages and some metabolism-revving recipes as well. If you stop losing weight or slow down, go back to a shake for lunch. Give it a try; you have nothing to lose but the pounds!

BREAKFAST
- High-quality whey protein shake made with water
- Black coffee or tea

SNACK
- Small apple

LUNCH
- High-quality whey protein shake made with water

SNACK
- Small apple (or any fruit from list) or legal snack

DINNER
- Choose 4 ounces of any lean protein from the list and a large salad with a minimum of 5 vegetables (10 is optimal) from the list

SNACK
- Anything from the legal snack list

QUICK TIPS

Men and Teens: Add one to two additional scoops of protein powder to your shakes or three to four egg whites. Or add an additional one to two ounces of fish to your meal plan to increase daily protein.

- **Still hungry?** Have more salad, vegetables, or clear broth; any of these will keep you satisfied and feeling full. A cup of tea or hot water with lemon works great after a meal too.
- **No alcohol or juice for the leanest results.**
- **Ideal Meal Times:** Breakfast at 7:00 a.m., snack at 10:00 a.m., lunch at 1:00 p.m., snack at 4:00 p.m., dinner at 7:00 p.m. No eating after 8: p.m.

Snack Options: A snack can satisfy head hunger and hold you over until your next meal. Snacks below boost your metabolism too.

- Cut-up veggies or garden salad with fat-free dressing
- Protein shake or protein bar
- Sugar-free, fat-free Jell-O or pudding
- Sugar-free, fat-free, low-calorie popsicle or Fudgesicle
- One serving (under 100 calories) fat-free low-sugar frozen yogurt or ice cream
- Air-popped popcorn (three cups) or 100-calorie bag Smart Food or microwave pop-corn.
- Small apple or half cup unsweetened or sugar-free applesauce (I like Musselman's)
- 100-calorie serving of almonds (about 8 to 10 nuts)
- Sugarless gum, menthol cough drops, Altoids, or fireballs help stop cravings.

THREE

Who Decides the Serving Size Anyway?

I've always told people that when it comes to portion size, "Don't blame me, I don't make the rules." While writing this book, I began to really wonder, who does decide? Who decides that one bottle will have two servings? That while the package comes with two pieces, it's only one serving? That 15 potato chips from the bag is how much you should eat at one time? Why does it seem so arbitrary sometimes? Figuring out serving sizes is a confusing issue—made more confusing by the ever-growing portion size in the United States. Can it be a coincidence that portions have grown larger every year and obesity rates have increased along with them (at an absurd rate, I might add)? If I may paraphrase Martha: Supersizing is not a good thing.

First of all, you need to know that portion and serving size are not the same thing. A portion is how much you put on your plate; a serving size is a measured specific amount of food that makes it easier for consumers to compare when buying. Portion and serving are similar, but not interchangeable. Health was not considered when coming up with serving size. It was created and ordered to be on food packages in 1994 as an industry standard, not to help you make smart food choices. When it comes to portions, you're supposed to figure that one out on your own.

Because there is so much confusion over what a true serving size is, there is no standard reference point for you to determine what is the appropriate amount of food to eat, let alone what you should be eating in the first place. Package labels differ so much from brand to brand that you cannot assume that a serving size of 15 chips per serving on a package of low-fat potato chips will be the same amount of food from one brand to the next. Guess what? It won't be.

Every day I have people crying out to me in despair, saying, "I have always been able to eat this food without gaining weight, but now when I eat it I gain five pounds immediately." Or "I track everything I eat in XYZ app, yet I still can't lose belly fat." Trying to find the reasons for this is a little bit harder than it used to be. You may think you're eating the right way, but you really aren't. It's getting harder to teach people the "whys" behind all these dilemmas, and that's because you have to pretty much unlearn what you've been taught about food portions and labels. Even I had to forget everything I had learned and start fresh. Only then did I begin to lose weight in spite of my slow metabolism.

> **LABELS, APPS, AND ONLINE DIET FITNESS PLANS ARE MORE LIKELY TO SABOTAGE YOU THAN HELP YOU LOSE WEIGHT.**

Before I get further into portion size and labels, you need to first understand these five weight loss truths:

1. After age 30, everything changes metabolically—you must accept that you need to do things differently to lose weight.
2. Every year of your life, your metabolism will slow down.
3. Whatever you think you're eating according to an app on your phone or PC is far off base. Use those apps as rough guides, not gospel. Did you know that these apps are allowed to be off by 20 percent in what they tell you? That's enough to stop weight loss and maybe even cause weight gain.
4. Your body needs only one-third of the food you eat every day for health and wellness. The other two-thirds is what you want to eat, not what you need.
5. Your belief system affects everything about your weight loss. If you don't believe something will work, you won't even try.

So what does this all have to do with serving sizes, you ask? Lots!

IT'S NOT YOUR FAULT

The most important thing I can teach you is that you need to take appropriate steps (like drinking a whey protein shake every day) to help offset these weight loss myths if you don't want to gain weight every year. Read the previous chapter, "Thermogenic Eating for Radical Weight Loss," again so you know which foods to eat and stick with them. Use the serving sizes and portions I recommend. And read labels carefully. I often spend time with clients showing them how label shenanigans affect their attempts at weight loss. And don't even get me started on weight loss apps. I have yet to find one I could recommend, even with reservations. They are the problem, not the solution. Eating too many calories and eating the wrong foods is what actually slows your metabolism.

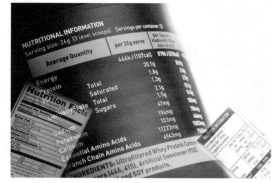

Don't be confused by labels that don't tell you what you need to know

Following the suggestions of labels and apps can lead you to stagnate, if not gain weight. I can tell you story after story about clients who spend far too much time arguing with me that they are eating perfectly, even meticulously, according to their apps or incredibly detailed computerized plans, yet still cannot lose weight or an inch of belly fat. If they only spent the time they spend arguing with me walking, they would be at goal weight or maybe even need to gain a few.

As much as it may sound like an excuse, the system really is at fault here. It's not you. Apps and labels can sabotage you. Do you know who sets the serving sizes you see on the side panel of your favorite food or on the computer diet and fitness program you use? You're going to be surprised. It's you. Well, people like you.

You might think that, in this day and age, labeling and servings would be determined by a more scientific approach. I always assumed that serving sizes were calculated to goals. So if you are trying to lose weight, you should eat this certain amount; but if you are trying to gain or maintain, it would be a different amount. Makes perfect sense that serving sizes should be different when you're a 6-foot-tall, 30-year-old man as opposed to a 4-foot-9-inch woman who is 55.

But how is it that growing children, teens, and people who are active are told to use the same serving sizes that you are using when trying to lose weight and shrink your waistline? Have you ever thought of it this way? Shouldn't serving sizes be a little bit different if you are tall or short or if you have lots of muscle or very little muscle? Ideally, shouldn't serving sizes factor in the rate you burn calories or take into account your metabolism's speed?

> SHOULDN'T SERVING SIZES BE A LITTLE DIFFERENT IF YOU ARE TALL OR SHORT OR IF YOU HAVE LOTS OF MUSCLE OR VERY LITTLE MUSCLE? IDEALLY, SHOULDN'T SERVING SIZES FACTOR IN THE RATE YOU BURN CALORIES AND TAKE INTO ACCOUNT YOUR METABOLISM'S SPEED?

I speak from my personal experience and the experiences of all the people I have helped over the years. Every time I tried to follow the food pyramid recommendations put forth by the U.S. government—and by the way, I was meticulous about serving sizes—I still gained weight. My metabolism is so slow that if I even look at half a serving of pasta, I gain five pounds; yet my 6-foot-tall and fairly active husband skips pasta at one meal and loses 10 pounds. (Okay, so that's a little bit of an exaggeration, but it sure feels like that's what happens.) I'm hoping this gets you thinking. You really have to be your own detective when it comes to losing weight.

Serving guidelines cannot serve as gospel, but merely as a rough gauge. The scale will show you every time if you're on the right track. If the scale isn't moving, you're still eating too much or eating the wrong foods for your metabolism. It's often a food you just can't let go of (a little cream in the coffee, perhaps?), but really need to. I urge you to follow my plan. It is guaranteed to work every time. Don't stop following these principles until you have lost all that fat you have hated for years. Your weight gain (or lack of weight loss) is not all your fault. Serving sizes (food choices, too) are mostly to blame, and I'm going to show you why.

PORTIONS VS. SERVINGS

According to the Cornell University Food and Brand Lab, (which is a great site full of very interesting information that I urge you to visit at foodpsychology.cornell.edu):

- Serving sizes have grown four times larger since 1950.
- Dinner plate size has grown 36 percent between 1960 and 2007.
- A serving of food served at home is now 33 percent larger than it was in 1996.
- Portion sizes can be two to eight times larger than USDA or FDA serving-size suggestions.
- The average woman has increased her weight by 24.5 pounds since 1950.
- The average man has increased his weight by 28.5 pounds since 1960.
- Chocolate chip cookies have quadrupled in size.
- The average pizza slice grew 70 percent in calories between 1982 and 2002.
- Caesar salads have doubled in calories.

The problem starts with who decides what and how much you should be eating. We are in trouble as a nation—we are, in fact, in the middle of an obesity epidemic that has reached crisis levels because the wrong people are deciding and telling us what a serving size should be. And guess who is making these decisions? WE are.

That's right; the serving size typically seen on nutrition labels (one slice of bread, 15 chips, 1 table-spoon of oil, an ounce or a quarter cup of almonds, 4 cookies, 100 grams, half a bottle, etc.) is de-termined by how much the typical American over the age of four consumes in a single sitting. Such questions were asked via national surveys, conducted in the 1970s and 1980s by the USDA Center for Nutrition Policy and Promotion, then averaged out and determined by federal researchers. (In 2005 this same group began updating those sizes.) That number was then rubber stamped on packages to make comparison shopping easier. It's not based on what you should eat, and it's not meant to be a suggestion of portion size. It's more of a simple gauge to aim for, with the assumption that you'll eat less if you're trying to lose weight.

I don't know about you, but even when I was little I ate more than the average American (I don't and never did have a shutoff valve or a body that knew intuitively when to stop). Or what about your obese neighbor who eats more for breakfast than she is supposed to eat in whole day? All of a sudden, a serving size can be skewed to something quite large. This isn't a good or scientific way to determine how to keep our weight within a healthy range. It's easy to see how we got into trouble in the first place, but that's only the beginning of the problem.

The first step you can take is realizing the suggested serving size is just that—suggested. It is not what you should consider the portion size. Serving size was created for manufacturers to hopefully create accurate and uniform nutrition labels across brands for comparison shopping. Use serving size as a rough gauge. Eat half or less of what's suggested. Can't stop eating once you start? Don't eat that particular food at all.

Even the director of the USDA Center for Nutrition Policy and Promotion, Dr. Robert Post, agrees. He has been quoted in several interviews, available online, stating: "You've got servings related to the nutrition facts panel, and then another issue is a reasonable portion of food to build a healthy eating pattern. That may be a little different. The serving size might be bigger than what we'd use in the nutrition world to promote good habits."

May be a little different? Might be bigger? How are you supposed to know this? When I turn around and try to teach people real portion size, I often get looks of disbelief, if not outright incredulous laughter. Seriously. I feel the same way. It's kind of a betrayal. You think you're eating right, reading labels, but you're still stuck and not losing weight.

The system needs to be fixed. Meanwhile, how do you make informed choices regarding your health and weight loss? The deeper issue that needs to be faced is that portions are out of control, and a serving size is often bigger than a portion. Serving size, portion … how are you supposed to know how much to eat? You need to adjust your portions, especially if you have more than 10 pounds to lose. You need to accept these metabolism-boosting laws as your weight-loss gospel. The worst thing that can happen to you when following this system is that you lose too much

WHAT TO KNOW ABOUT LABELS AND SERVING SIZE

To keep your metabolism running at optimal speeds and keep the weight off, you need to remember this:

- The serving sizes you see on a Nutrition Facts Panel are based on servings commonly eaten, and they are not necessarily recommended. The serving sizes on a label are standardized so that you should be able to compare one product to another—a slice of bread from one brand to another. They are nothing more than a tool with which to compare different brands and versions of the same product.
- Always look at the label so that you know how many calories and other nutrients are in the package that you purchased, but don't use it as a guide for how much to eat. Eat at most half of what you think you should or don't eat it at all.
- Assume that all packages are more than one serving.
- When in doubt, don't eat it. If you have to ask yourself, you already know the answer.

weight too fast. Wouldn't that be awful?

Fast weight loss isn't unhealthy when you follow *The Metabolism Solution*. My program is full of health-generating nutrition compared to incorrect and un-balanced diets that lack protein or deny all carbohydrates. The only carbs you should be afraid of are the ones that have labels on them. Vegetables are the only food that we under-eat.

IF YOU CAN'T PORTION CONTROL A CERTAIN FOOD, DON'T EAT IT!

When it comes to figuring out how much you should be eating, think of yourself like the gas tank of a car. If the tank holds only 10 gallons, then you can put in only 10 gallons, period. It doesn't matter how slow or fast your metabolism is. The limit is the limit. Doesn't matter how high-end the gasoline is either (or how healthy the food is), you cannot add more than the tank holds. You can only add more gasoline when you burn up some of the gas already in your tank. Does that make sense?

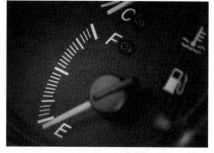

Are you overfilling your "gas tank" with food?

PORTIONS, SERVINGS, AND THE METABOLISM SOLUTION

How do I know how many "servings" of vegetables and fruit are right for me?
You want to find your right balance. For instance, if you are five feet tall and slight of frame, you will likely need fewer total servings of food than someone that might be over six feet tall and very active. There are plenty of professional recommendations out there as to what you "should" eat. Consider that this is not about finding the right rules, but rather choosing foundational principles to live by for your own optimal health. You know what works by what the scale shows. Keeping track of your body weight and journaling exactly what and how much you eat is critical so you can see cause and effect on the scale and know which foods you need to cut.

Why do you recommend so many servings of vegetables?
In the world of nutritional science, scientists might disagree about which foods are best to consume, but all agree that vegetables (preferably organic) are good for you. These recommendations are based on the fact that vegetables (especially green leafy ones) are the best way to lose belly fat. Vegetables are delicious, nutritional powerhouses that stimulate the fat-burning process and keep you healthy.

If white fish is so healthy, why can't I eat as much as I want?
Your body can only digest a certain amount of protein from each meal (a rough gauge puts it at approximately 24 to 30 grams). Any excess you eat—no matter how healthy—is stored as fat to be used later. This occurs when overeating any type of protein, even a lean, clean protein like white fish. Remember the gas tank analogy? If you're five feet tall, your gas tank is totally different from the one your six-foot-tall husband has. If you eat the same amount, even though your husband's gas tank is larger, you gain weight no matter how fast your metabolism is. It's very simple; eat only what you need, and you lose weight every time. Not losing? You're eating more than you're burning. I know it's brutal, but it's honest; and the sooner you accept this, the faster you'll lose weight. Don't beat yourself up when you overeat, just jump back on the plan or drink more shakes the next day instead of fussing over what to eat, when, or how much and dealing with the portion struggle.

What's the best way to find my portion size?
How do you know if your portions are too big? You weigh them using a food scale. Don't guess, and don't trust your eye. Weigh the food you eat.

So how do you figure out a label and know portion size? For the fastest and easiest road to weight loss, follow the serving and portion sizes in this book. Weigh and measure everything that goes into your mouth. Make a game out of it; it's not a punishment.

Many of these portion sizes are going to seem small, if not downright tiny. I'm not particularly fond of them either. But I also know that in order to lose weight you need to abide by God's laws and learn to eat to fill your body's gas tank. Be honest and stop making excuses. Even "I only ate a little!" can sabotage you. Excuses are like telling your 10-gallon gas tank why it's okay that you're trying to squeeze in 15 gallons. You know what happens—the excess gas pours out all over the car no matter how expensive the gas is. Unfortunately, the excess food we eat doesn't just dribble away off our bodies.

If you are in the category of those trying to lose those last 10 pounds, you need to be even more careful about the amount of fuel you put in your car! Make sure that every ounce of fuel is carefully measured and accounted for, follow *the Metabolism Solution* eating plan exactly as specified, and I promise you that you will start to see the scale moving!

Knowing your numbers (food portions and calories, for example) is the way to boost your metabolism and lose weight for good. But better yet is eating food that doesn't come with labels. Avoid the foods with labels, and you won't have to determine what a reasonable portion size is for yourself. Eat fresh foods from the earth as much as you can. And if you are reading labels, always go for less than the serving size suggestion states. Once you have reached your goals following *The Metabolism Solution* to a T, then—and only then—you can slowly and cautiously try adding back some of the foods you love. Just never stop drinking a whey protein shake for breakfast.

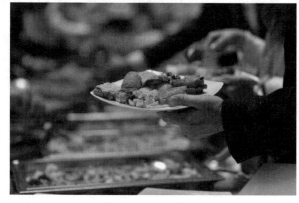

All you can eat? No way!

You almost need a Ph.D. in label science or a nutritionist on speed dial to really comprehend what or how much you're supposed to eat. To keep the weight off, keep it simple and stick to fish and lots of veggies.

WHAT HAS REPLACED THE FOOD PYRAMID?

If you're carrying extra weight, scoring high on the BMI chart, and your scale is telling you to lose a few or more than a few, then your portion sizes are too big. Portions have become supersized over the years, and most people no longer know how much food they are actually shoveling into their mouths.

Knowing the proper portion size can help stop you from packing on extra calories as well as extra pounds.

The decision of when and what to eat should be based on what your body needs, not what you feel like. The quantity of food you choose should always be based on your age, gender (males and growing children may need more than females), your level of physical activity, body mass index, and what you're about to do. For example, if you're going to bed, you really can skip the food as your body is going to sleep and doesn't need many calories to do so. Now, if you are going to the gym or about to move furniture around, your body may need some extra calories. If you don't overfeed your body, you'll end up burning excess fat as fuel instead of your last meal.

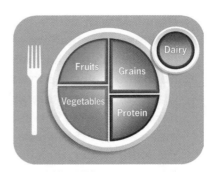

USDA Dinner Plate Guide

Keep in mind that if you are 20 pounds or more overweight, you won't starve if you don't eat a lot before a workout or higher activity levels. If your total body fat measures at 10 percent or under, you need to add calories before a workout to keep your body from chewing up muscle. But if you're over 10 percent body fat (and most of us are), you don't need to worry.

In 2011, the U.S. Department of Agriculture replaced the older food pyramid (we were actually less overweight when the food pyramid was designed) with a new symbol that dictates the recommended servings for each food group. The new food guide is called "The Dinner Plate." As its name would indicate, this is a dish-shaped icon, divided into five sections and labeled with the essential food groups: fruits, vegetables, grains, proteins, and dairy. This breakdown of types of foods to eat may be fine for those maintaining, but for those trying to lose weight, it doesn't work.

How do you know if foods affect you differently or slow your metabolism? You just know. Try this little self-test: What are the five foods that come to mind right now? Most likely they are the ones you wonder if you'll be able to eat; these are most likely the ones you should avoid. Abstaining is easier than fighting with food if you can't control your portions. Try it, you'll see. The one thing I agree with the USDA on is that vegetables should take up the majority of your plate. I say even more than the new plate depicts. The new guidelines also stress adding more "color" to your dish, and there is no better way to do this than eating your veggies. Color and texture are critical because we eat with all of our senses and vegetables provide both.

THESE WORDS MAY NOT MEAN WHAT YOU THINK THEY MEAN

IF IT SAYS "WHOLE GRAIN"—REFRAIN. All grains start their lives as whole grains, complete with a fully intact seed that includes three separate components. However, refining grains tends to remove the two outermost parts of the seed, stripping much of the grain's protein and at least 17 key nutrients. Whole grains have some protein, fiber, and many important vitamins and minerals that refined grains often lack. "Whole Grain" on a label means that it must have the same amount of all three seed components as a freshly harvested kernel. Words like bran, wheat germ, and fiber do not mean a product is whole grain. Check the ingredients. If the first ingredient contains the word whole, then it's likely (though not guaranteed) that the product is mostly whole grain. If only the second ingredient contains the word whole, then the product may contain anywhere from 1 to 49 percent whole grain. With multigrain breads, it can be even harder to know how much of it is truly whole grain. If you want to be completely confident that you're eating whole grains, look for a Whole Grain Stamp. If a product has a 100% Stamp, then all the grain ingredients are whole grains, and it contains at least a full serving (16 grams) of whole grains. A Basic Stamp means the product has at least 8 grams (a half serving) of whole grains, though it may also have refined grains.

"CHOLESTEROL-FREE" DOESN'T MEAN GOOD FOR YOU OR GOOD FOR WEIGHT LOSS. Cholesterol is naturally found in foods like red meat (yes, even lean chicken has some), dairy, egg yolks, and fish (shellfish mostly, not white fish). Research now suggests that eating foods that naturally contain cholesterol may not contribute to high blood cholesterol levels as much as was once thought. Many foods that are labeled cholesterol-free never would have contained cholesterol to begin with—but labeling them this way can trick you into thinking you're buying something healthy. It's more important to look at fat and calories—and especially sugars.

"NOW WITH LESS FAT"—AND YOU'LL STILL GAIN WEIGHT. Foods advertised as being "reduced fat" contain at least 25 percent less fat than a similar reference food does. However, less fat can mean less flavor and less satisfaction, and you might wind up eating more because you think you can. Manufacturers often try to make up for this lack of flavor satisfaction by adding sugar and sodium. You may be tempted to eat more of the reduced-fat food, leaving you with a bigger waistline than if you stuck with the original and ate a little less.

"ZERO TRANS FATS" DOES NOT MEAN YOU WON'T GAIN FAT. Trans fats are a dangerous type of fat often used in baked goods, frozen foods, frostings, coffee creamers, and microwave popcorns, among many other foods. They are a major contributor to weight gain and heart disease and have already been banned or eliminated from many foods and restaurants. But beware: Current labeling guidelines allow manufacturers to say that any food that contains less than 0.5 grams of trans fats per serving contains "Zero Trans Fats." Even small amounts of these fats (like the amount you splash into your coffee everyday) can add up over time to severely damage your blood vessels and heart—not to mention make you gain weight by slowing down your metabolism. To make sure you're avoiding trans fats entirely, watch out for foods that list partially hydrogenated oil, hydrogenated vegetable oil, and shortening on their ingredients list. These foods contain trans fats.

"LIGHTLY SALTED" DOESN'T MEAN IT WON'T MAKE YOU RETAIN WATER OR GAIN WATER WEIGHT. If a food says it is "lightly salted," that generally means that it has 50 percent less sodium than the amount in a similar reference food, which does not necessarily make it low in sodium. To keep track of how much salt you're actually eating, check the amount of sodium on the label and try to stay under 2,300 mg a day. People with certain health conditions may need to stick to low-sodium foods, which contain no more than 140 mg of sodium per serving. Retaining water is the reason the scale can go up so fast. Eat more asparagus and drink more water to offset that water retention, and you'll be fine by day's end. A good, sweaty workout doesn't hurt, either.

SELL-BY DATES. Terms like "sell by," "use by," and "best before" are usually not good indicators of how safe the food is to eat. Rather than referring to when the food is safe to eat, these terms are simply suggestions from the manufacturer for when the food is at its peak quality. The "sell by" date tells grocery stores how long to offer the product for sale, and food is usually fresh for at least several days after that date. "Best by" usually speaks to when the food has its best flavor and quality. "Use by" is the last date recommended for use of the product at its peak quality. Confusion over these dates prompts nine out of ten Americans to throw away food before they really need to—a waste of taste and money. Freezing foods changes all of this. Freeze your protein bars and they last forever. Just remember to thaw them out before trying to bite into one.

DECODING THE FOOD LABEL

Let's get back to labels. Remember that just because you paid a lot for a food or the label says that it's "100% All Natural" and good for you does not mean it is good for weight loss. These so-called health halo foods such as whole grain and reduced fat foods may not be what you think and are most often the reason we struggle with our weight. Marketers want us to believe we need to eat these foods, when in fact we don't.

Did you know that food labels often advertise healthy promises on the outside that the food on the inside may not keep? Learn which labels require a closer look with this easy-to-understand guide. I'm not actually suggesting that you eat these foods, but I want you to know what they mean should you decide to indulge or justify on your food journal that what you ate was healthy. And don't assume these foods won't affect your weight loss. This couldn't be further from the truth.

There are so many misconceptions out there when it comes to food and weight loss. The idea that cheeses, peanut butter, nuts, and yogurt are good sources of protein is one that comes to mind. Or maybe you were one of the unlucky ones that saw on TV how avocados could help you shrink your thighs because they contain a "good" fat? While these foods may contain some nutrients like protein or fats, they aren't the best sources of protein, and the fats aren't essential; therefore, these foods aren't the best for weight loss. You usually need to overeat them to get the nutrients you need, and unless you are extremely physically active, (even I don't qualify) you'd be getting more calories than you need so they would cause weight gain or, at the very least, stop your weight loss.

You know slacking on exercise, not drinking enough water, or not getting enough sleep slows weight loss. But another big culprit is falling off the eating plan, be it for a weekend, one day, or even for a meal. When cheating, you might eat too much of a food you shouldn't, or you may not pay meticulous attention to what and how much you are supposed to eat when following *The Metabolism Solution*. Then there's one of the most serious threats to weight loss: eating out.

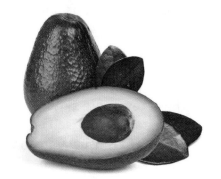

When we eat out, we tend to slip up on rich dressings and toppings like grated cheese, bacon bits, and croutons. You burn 300 calories by walking for three miles, but when you eat a 300-calorie muffin while meeting a friend for coffee, you totally erase the effect of your workout. It can happen so fast and without much thought on your part.

The Metabolism Solution is a healthy, calorie-controlled meal plan that's complete with exercise to help maximize calorie burning and encourage permanent weight control. But if you blow off the rules, even one meal off the plan, you can trash a whole week's worth of effort. Don't think you can be lax with your calories because you exercise, and don't become lax about exercise just because you're cutting calories. Keep the following in mind the next time you say, "I only ate a little!" It's still too much.

Want to know what else may be stopping your weight loss? Eating foods that are higher in carbs, sugars, and fats than you think they are. Below are my rules for decoding labels.

THE FOOD LABEL READING RULES

Rule #1. If it's not on *The Metabolism Solution* food list, it is not good for weight loss even though it may be good for you.

Rule #2. Don't pay any attention to those marketing claims on the front of the food packages. What the back label says counts most. The front of a label is created to sell, not educate. The back is where the truth lies.

Rule #3. The highest number listed on the back label is what determines what nutrient category that food falls under because it contains the most of that nutrient. So if a food is a source of whey protein, whey protein should be the highest number you see listed on the label.

Guess which food I'm talking about here. According to its label, it is a health food, yet it stops you from losing weight—not because it's bad for you, but because it's one of those "jack of all trades, master of none" foods. Is it a protein? A carbohydrate? Something else? Millions of dieters enjoy it every day for breakfast or lunch and still don't see their waistlines shrinking. Are you wondering what that food is? It's yogurt. Don't get me wrong—yogurt has a place in our lives; I eat it just about every day, but as a healthy dessert. Why a dessert? It doesn't have enough protein to qualify for a metabolic-boosting meal and has too much sugar. As a dessert it delivers some nutrition and satisfies me.

	Nonfat Greek Yogurt	Protein Bar	Sports Drink
Serving Size	150 g	50 g	500 ml
Calories	100	180	120
Fat Calories	0	40	0
Total Fat	0	4.5 g	0
Saturated Fat	0	3 g	0
Protein	12 g	20 g	0
Cholesterol	10 mg	15 mg	0
Total Carbs	14 g	17 g	29 g
Fiber	<1 g	2 g	0
Sugar	13 g	2 g	29 g

Any time you are confused about calories and wonder if you should reach for a certain food, ask yourself the following questions:

1. How many servings are in the container and can you stop at one portion?
2. How many grams of protein does it contain per serving? Keep in mind a perfect serving of protein is between 20 and 24 grams. In order to be considered a protein source, the food needs to have that amount.
3. How much sugar does it contain per serving? Look for all sugars—including sugar from agave, honey, or any and all natural sources. All sugars count. Aim for none or the lowest number you can find. Splenda and Truvia don't count because they won't affect your insulin levels.
4. How many carbohydrates does it contain per serving? Aim for the lowest carbs possible: less than 20 grams per serving unless it's a leafy green vegetable. If it is above 20 grams, it is a carb and should be limited.
5. How much fat does it contain per serving? Aim for the lowest number possible and don't eat the food if it contains more than five grams of fat per serving—unless it's salmon.

Of course, calories count. Check to see how many calories the food item contains and do the math for each serving, counting calories and grams, to make sure you do not go over your daily requirement. IF you follow the above rules, it brings the calories down for you.

TOP NINE FOOD SINS YOU CAN AVOID IF YOU READ THE LABELS

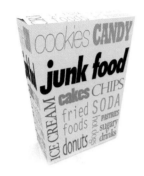

Food sins don't make you thin!

Now we're down to the nitty-gritty. The foods listed here, even if you have only a little bit of them, will affect your metabolism. It's not just about calories but the metabolic effect that these foods have on our waistlines because they trigger an insulin response that stops weight loss every time. And many of these foods tend to trigger the same part of our brain that drugs do (the addiction center), so we become addicted and usually eat too much.

Even though you exercise and make sure there is enough room in your plan for it calorically, these foods will sabotage your weight loss. Unfortunately, you can't count on your smartphone app to run all your numbers for you because those apps can be significantly off. You won't get lean if you take the caloric numbers from these apps as your gospel. You need to make a concerted effort to avoid the following food sins in order to experience real weight loss success on *The Metabolism Solution*.

Food Sin #1: Feta Cheese, the "Low-Fat" Cheese

One tiny little cube (about the size of a die) contains 6 grams of fat. Who eats just one cube? With 15 grams of fat allowed per day on *The Metabolism Solution* plan, you had better not be adding any other fats to your meals if you reach for the cheese. I love cheese, but it is best used for weight-gain diets. That's the only time I suggest it, (except for reduced-fat Parmesan cheese). If you're serious about losing weight, skip the cheese.

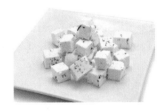

Food Sin #2: Oils

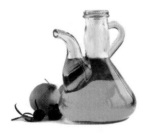

The 15-grams-of-fat-a-day rule is very important when it comes to losing weight and fat especially. One tablespoon of oil has 120 calories and 14 grams of fat. Doesn't leave much fat to have the rest of the day, does it? Even if you use a little, it's probably still too much. Use sprays or learn how to use chicken broth in cooking and stick to vinegar on your salads. Salad dressings will undo all the work you do by eating those healthy vegetables. You can't lose body fat if you keep eating lots of fats, even the "good ones." You'll continuously be replenishing your fat supply before you can burn what you already have.

Food Sin #3: Ice Cream

The serving size for ice cream is one half cup. Who eats only that much? Who can't go through a pint of ice cream in one sitting? That one recommended serving will set you back 250 calories, 13 grams of fat, and 30 carbohydrates, all of which come from sugar. Even one tablespoon is enough to set you back. If you absolutely have to indulge, and you are committed to losing weight, go for low-fat, sugar-free frozen yogurt. That is my true indulgence.

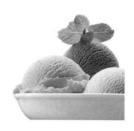

Food Sin #4: Peanut Butter

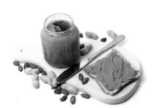

Peanut butter is a dieter's worst enemy because it is so deceptive. Most women eat one tablespoon of it straight out of the jar. In two tablespoons (the serving recommendation), you get 17 grams of fat and only 8 grams of protein. More grams of fat than protein. Guess what? It's a fat, and stop calling it anything else. Stop licking that peanut butter spoon, and you can lose eight pounds in a year—it's that big a deal. Quit eating peanut butter altogether and lose even more weight. Peanut butter is best for underweight hikers who need to eat a lot of calories. It's not good for the metabolism because it is not a complete protein and contains too much fat. Remember our 15-grams-of-fat-a-day rule?

Food Sin #5: Coffee Creamer, AKA That Dash of Milk

This was the hardest thing for me to give up. No matter how little you use or how "insignificant" you may feel the amount is, it can hold you back from your weight loss goals. Do a test and see for yourself. The scale will tell all. It's not about the calories but where they come from, and this stuff is made of fat and sugar. All that fat and sugar in creamers can't make muscle or nourish eyes, skin, or hair. There isn't one nutritious ingredient in there. Your body is left

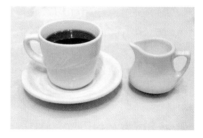

wondering, "What do you want me to do with this stuff?" So guess where it goes? Straight to your hips, thighs, and belly. Giving it up is worth it when you see how much better you look and feel and how much time you save in the gym.

Food Sin #6: Bread and Pasta

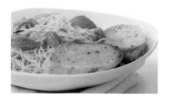

These two tie for sixth place. Bread and pasta are nothing more than empty carbs that will need to be burned off in the gym. If you're serious about losing weight, stay away from these high-carb, high-calorie foods. Even at their recommended serving size, they are over the limit in carbs and calories. Can you stick to one portion? One slice of bread (hope you like open-faced sandwiches) or a half-cup of cooked pasta? (Remember, the portion is often smaller than the recommended serving size). In a two-ounce serving as recommended by some pasta labels (Who even knows how much that is? Do you?), you get at least 200 calories and 35 to 40 carbohydrates per serving. Some pastas even have fat. It would take you one hour to burn that off in the gym—and that's if you only ate one portion. Bread is a metabolic nightmare. It doesn't matter how healthy or artisanal it is or how much you paid for it. Limit it, and you'll lose faster; it truly is that simple. Bread can set you back 21 carbs and 170 calories per slice (and some breads recommend two slices per serving). No matter how much protein a bread label may claim, it will always have more carbs. Bread can never be a protein. It is a carb. Look at the labels. Look at all the sugar. Notice that the carb number is significantly larger than the protein number? Breads are almost always diet deceivers. Giving up bread will move that dial on the scale. I guarantee it.

Food Sin #7: Yogurt

Ah, yogurt. I love the stuff. Yogurt, like most dairy, is an incomplete protein, loaded with sugar, fats, and all kinds of unknowns that slow your metabolism. I've managed to keep it in my diet by treating it as a dessert. I can't tell you how many stories I hear from people telling me how they struggle in trying to lose weight. Guess what they're eating for breakfast? Some so-called sugar-free, healthy yogurt. Yes, nonfat, sugar-free yogurt is better than ice cream, but it is never going to be a complete protein and will never beat a high-quality whey protein for title of Metabolic-Boosting Breakfast.

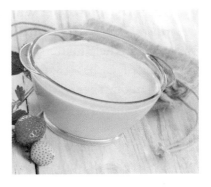

I have a kid's size yogurt just about every day as dessert from my local frozen yogurt place. It keeps me feeling full and satisfied, and I don't feel like I'm on a diet. In fact, ever since I started this habit, I have never been more on track with my eating in my life. I feel alive and part of the world—and I don't

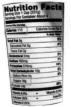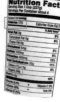 miss ice cream anymore. In this day and age, there are all kinds of frozen yogurt stands no matter where you are. Aim for the smallest size available, and if it's self-serve, simply count "one Mississippi, two Mississippi, three Mississippi," and you should get a three-ounce portion. Always look for the lowest calories and sugar, and make sure it's nonfat so it is cleanest and won't slow your metabolism.

Take a look at the labels. A small serving of a so-called healthy high-protein yogurt has 33 grams of carbohydrates, and it's all from sugar—that's 8 ¼ teaspoons of sugar. Most yogurt labels also specify 0 grams of fat, but the ingredients list states it is made from whole milk solid, which definitely has fat.

Food Sin #8: Pizza

I have never met anyone who can eat just one slice of pizza. Every Monday morning, I hear at least one of my clients complaining about lack of weight loss, only to admit it was pizza night on Friday. Pizza is better for weight gain and never works for weight loss. Your favorite pie is one of the highest calorie foods per ounce, full of fats and carbs. Don't buy into the claim that you're getting all your food groups or that it's loaded with vegetables so it's healthy. Avoid pizza. The vegetables on it may be healthy on their own, if they're not pre-pared in fat, but not when smothered in cheese and placed on bread. The meats usually found on pizza are far too high in fat to count as 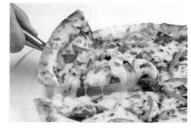 sufficient protein to offset the carbs and fats already in the pizza. How many times have you blotted your pepperoni pizza slice before eating it? Think that's good for weight loss?

I can hear you from here: What about moderation? If you're at goal and doing fine maintaining, then every now and then (and limiting yourself to two slices) might be okay. But if you are struggling, pizza isn't going to help matters. Two plain cheese slices will set you back 740 calories, 36 grams of fat, and 72 grams of carbs—that's more than two days' worth of fat and carbs and three extra hours at the gym. Even one slice is too much. Yes, even thin crust pizza. Did you know that thin crust is just as high in carbohydrates? It's just rolled thinner. Don't think of thin crust pizza as a low-calorie alternative. It's not.

Food Sin #9: Alcohol

They may grow the grapes in California, but I think Fairfield County in Connecticut is the wine-drinking capital of the United States. I run into so many people who defend their nightly glass of Merlot and refuse to take it out of their diet—all while ranting about how they just can't lose those last few pounds or that spare tire around the middle. Wine has nutritional value, they argue, containing minerals and antioxidants. But so do vegeta-bles—and more of them. Wine is a big factor, especially when it comes to belly fat. Why is that? Because alcohol has almost two times the amount of carbs and sugars. Wine is a carbohydrate full of empty calories. A glass of wine can contain from nine to nineteen grams of carbs per serving; 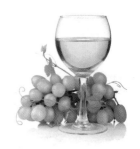 flavored wines can have even more. And who follows the serving size when pouring a glass? Do you even know what it is?

In some cases a slightly sweet and low-alcohol wine may have fewer calories than a dry, high-alcohol wine. But you'd be hard pressed to know for sure since wine doesn't come with labels. Neither do other kinds of alcohol. No calorie counts, no grams of carbohydrates—not even serving suggestions. And guess why? Because wine and liquors are not considered part of a daily diet. They are not required to disclose nutritional information by law. Perhaps labels should be required? You can dig around to find calorie and "nutritional" information, but it would be much easier if it were on the bottle.

When it comes to a glass of wine, which is a 6-ounce serving, calories can range anywhere from just over 100 (for a sweet white wine low in alcohol) to almost 300 (for a sweet dessert wine). Popular types like Merlot and Chardonnay tend to fall in the 150-to-200-calorie range per glass. When it comes to your daily calories, would you rather eat a salad loaded with vegetables that will fill you up or have a glass of wine that will leave you hungry?

> WHEN IT COMES TO YOUR DAILY CALORIES, WOULD YOU RATHER EAT A SALAD LOADED WITH VEGETABLES THAT WILL FILL YOU UP OR HAVE A GLASS OF WINE THAT WILL LEAVE YOU HUNGRY?

The bottom line is that it is the quality of your calories that counts. Remember: better is better. You want to take in calories that will boost your metabolism, not just fill you up. This is oh-so-especially important when you're trying to lose belly fat. Empty calories (processed foods are mostly empty calories) have no job to do; thus, they store as fat very easily compared to the clean food plan of *The Metabolism Solution*. Want to know where empty calories go? They go straight to your hips, thighs, and belly. I know that you want to get rid of the extra fat in those areas. Try eliminating these "food sins" from your diet and watch what happens. I dare you!

FOUR

Irresistibly Delicious Thermogenic Recipes

I know that after two chapters of hearing about which thermogenic foods are allowed on *The Metabolism Solution* and what foods to avoid, you are probably wondering what your meals are going to look like and what you will be cooking, right? I have some great news for you: Incorporating healthy, clean foods into your diet is not only good for you, it's delicious!

After 13 years with Martha Stewart, I've learned a thing or two about cooking. Anyone can cook with butter and oil. The true art form is to create tasty dishes without them. Did you know that professional chefs practice a new recipe at least 10 times before they get it just right? Practice until you get it right.

Now that you have been armed with the knowledge of the thermogenic foods you need to eat for weight loss, wouldn't you like to prepare some mouth-watering meals using them? The following pages contain the recipes I use to satisfy and de-fatify. Some of them may seem familiar, as I've taken several comfort-food-type dishes, including some of my childhood favorites, and remade them, thermogenic-style.

That doesn't mean these recipes are low on flavor. Each recipe is Weight Watchers-, Paleo-, and South Beach-friendly and, more importantly, meets *The Metabolism Solution* requirements: low-calorie, low-carb, very low-fat, low-sodium, and gluten-free, while packing in all the good stuff—fiber, protein, and beneficial nutrients to boost your metabolism. It's food so healthy even your doctor will approve. And the best part? It's absolutely delightful for your taste buds. Your family will think you took a cooking class—all that for under 300 calories a meal.

Use the foods, condiments, and spices on the lists to make your favorite meals thermogenic. When you're pressed for time, search for store-bought ingredients with the lowest calories, fats, and carbs. Be careful when it comes to sugar, too; so many foods—especially sauces and dressings—are loaded with it. Sometimes you need to shop around until you find a store-bought brand that meets your weight-loss needs and tastes great.

CHICKEN AND TURKEY

Cooking lean protein is very different from preparing red or fatty meat. Because they are lower in fat, chicken and turkey can dry out quickly; because they are also lower in sodium, you'll need to add additional spices to get the flavor your taste buds crave. You can always add water, broth, or a low-fat sauce to any recipe to make your poultry more moist.

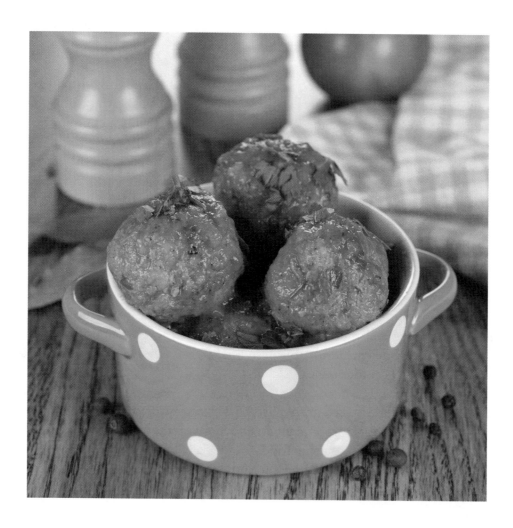

POPPA VINNIE'S TURKEY MEATBALLS

Minutes to Prepare: 20 • Minutes to Cook: 40 • Number of Servings: 6

I know every cook claims to make the best meatballs, but none compare to my Grandfather Vinnie's. Don't tell my mom: I've modified his original recipe, using turkey instead of beef and baking instead of frying to make it low-fat. You will not find a better, leaner meatball. I enjoy these on top of a bed of broccoli along with a green salad. You can modify the recipe to create turkey burgers as well.

> 1 lb. 97% lean ground turkey
> 3 garlic cloves, minced
> ¼ cup onion, finely chopped
> ¼ cup parsley, chopped
> ½ teaspoon pepper
> ½ teaspoon oregano
> 2 egg whites, beaten
> ½ cup dry Italian seasoned breadcrumbs
> 1 tablespoon fennel seeds (optional)

Always sauté your onions and garlic first, then mix all the ingredients and shape into 30 meatballs, approximately 1 inch across. Place meatballs on a nonstick baking pan that's been lightly sprayed with olive oil and bake at 350 degrees for 15 minutes. Turn them once and cook for another 25 minutes. Cooking times may vary—keep your eyes on these precious meatballs so they don't burn. Once browned, you can always throw them into your sauce and cook them for an additional 10 to 15 minutes until cooked through.

GAETANO'S CHICKEN SCARPIELLO

Minutes to Prepare: 10 to 15 • Minutes to Cook: 10 to 15 • Number of Servings: 4

This was my Great-Uncle Guy's (Gaetano's) family recipe. I make this in a flash, and it appeals to all the senses. It tastes even better the next day—if you have any leftovers. Try it over a salad or make it the filling for lettuce tacos. You can cook this on a grill or in tinfoil for easier cleanup. You can also make this on a George Foreman Grill by adding the peppers on top of the chicken breast. Want something different for cheat night? Make this with turkey sausage—but be sure to buy the leanest you can find. I like Jennie-O's.

    4 4- to 5-oz. chicken breasts
    1 large red pepper, sliced or 1 cup frozen
    1 large green pepper, sliced or 1 cup frozen
    1 large yellow or orange pepper, sliced or 1 cup frozen
    1 to 2 large onions, sliced (frozen is fine)
    ½ teaspoon oregano
    1 small bottle of sliced hot cherry peppers and juice
    NoSalt and pepper to taste
    1 tablespoon chopped garlic
    Olive oil spray

Grill or broil chicken breast in oven or use precooked and warmed. In a large skillet, sprayed with olive oil spray, sauté garlic, onions, peppers, oregano, NoSalt, and pepper until partially cooked. (Add water or defatted chicken stock if you need more liquid so it doesn't get too dry.)

Cut chicken into bite-size pieces and combine with peppers and onions. Stir in hot peppers and juice and continue to cook 10 to 15 minutes or until chicken is fork tender—be careful not to overcook.

EASY ITALIAN PORTOBELLO CHICKEN WITH RED ONIONS

Minutes to Prepare: 5 • Minutes to Cook: 12 • Number of Servings: 1

It's no secret that I like to eat—and I like to eat a lot. I'm not proud of it, but luckily I have found a way to eat a lot and lose a lot, too. That's why this filling combo is good for you and your metabolism. I love chicken, but I just don't lose easily when I eat a lot of it. Mixing it with Portobello mushrooms is a good trick to fill you up while introducing different colors and textures to your diet.

½ precooked sliced chicken breast
1 Portobello mushroom
½ red onion, sliced
Olive oil spray
Balsamic vinegar
NoSalt and Pepper

Preheat oven to 425 degrees. Remove stem from mushroom cap, spray cap with olive oil and place stem side up on rimmed baking sheet or pan. Sprinkle lightly with NoSalt and pepper. Bake 15 minutes or until mushroom is hot. Slice Portobello into long slices.

While mushroom bakes, sauté onions in a pan lightly sprayed with olive oil or grill lightly on a George Foreman Grill. When onion is translucent, add mushroom and chicken slices along with balsamic vinegar and continue cooking until all is heated through.

Garlic and Lime Chicken Breast

Minutes to Prepare: 10 to 15   •   Minutes to Cook: 25 to 30   •   Number of Servings: 4

Do you crave Mexican food but don't want to blow your diet? You can add 1 tsp. of chili powder or a few shakes of hot sauce for more zing. Eating this dish can save you thousands of calories and help you melt fat instead of gaining it. This is what my family eats when we want Mexican flavor. It's a great dish for company, too. I like to serve this with a chopped salad that's topped with a mixture of cucumbers, sweet onions, and tomatoes chopped salsa-style, sprinkled with NoSalt and pepper, drizzled with a little bit of lime juice and two to three squirts of spray olive oil. This dish can be cooked in tinfoil or on the grill for easy cleanup. For a quick appetizer, make extra salad topping to use as a dip for cucumber slices while you wait for dinner. Try the marinade for shrimp or as a dressing.

¼ cup fresh or bottled lime juice
1 tablespoon olive oil
⅓ cup defatted chicken broth (look for gluten-, MSG-, and soy-free if possible)
1 tablespoon minced garlic (jarred is fine)
4 (5-oz.) boneless, skinless chicken breast halves

Preheat oven to 400 degrees. In a large bowl, whisk together lime juice, oil, broth, and garlic. Season generously with NoSalt and pepper. Add chicken, turning to coat. If possible, marinate chicken, covered and chilled, turning once or twice, at least two hours and up to one day.

Remove chicken from marinade and arrange, without crowding, in a shallow baking pan. Season with NoSalt and pepper and roast in oven until just cooked through, 25 minutes or less depending on your oven. Do not overcook. (Before cooking, drizzle with leftover marinade and bake covered for more moist chicken.)

Serve with chopped salad, green beans, and baby roasted carrots.

GRANDMA MARY'S CHICKEN POTACCIO
(CHICKEN WITH RED WINE VINEGAR AND VEGETABLES)

Minutes to Prepare: 10 • Minutes to Cook: 20 • Serves: 4

This is one of the best home-cooked chicken dishes ever. My grandma prepared it, and anything she made seemed like it was cooked with love and tasted dreamy. I can remember walking into her house, and it smelled heavenly. Now you know how I learned that food was love. Be sure to make extra, as this dish tastes even better the day after. This recipe works great and is much faster with small chicken cutlets or strips, shrimp, or fish—just adjust the cooking time and amount of spice as needed. Mangia!

4 medium boneless, skinless chicken breasts (cut-up frying chicken works for a family)
2 tablespoons rosemary leaves
1 teaspoon olive oil
7 tablespoons chicken broth
10 garlic cloves, peeled
½ cup red wine vinegar
NoSalt and pepper, optional

In a large frying pan with a tight cover, heat olive oil and chicken broth. Add chicken, NoSalt, and pepper, stirring often and cooking chicken to a nice golden brown. Add garlic, rosemary, and vinegar. Lower heat, cover, and simmer gently for 15 to 20 minutes.

When chicken is fork tender, remove cover and turn up the heat to reduce liquid in pan. You can always add more water or chicken broth for additional liquid so chicken doesn't get dry. Keep in mind, there is no fat in this recipe, so liquids may need to be added back in. Stir chicken pieces until well coated in pan juices.

Serve with sautéed escarole or green beans and, of course, always with a salad.

POPPA JIM'S CHICKEN TETRAZZINI

Minutes to Prepare: 20 • Minutes to Cook: 30 to 40 • Serves: 4

My father loved to cook, and Chicken Tetrazzini was one of his favorites. Now that he is gone, I find myself wanting to make his favorites as a way to be close to him.

4 (4-oz.) boneless, skinless chicken breasts
1 cup or more of fat-free chicken broth
⅔ cup or less of condensed evaporated skim milk (omit for a leaner meal)
1 lb. mushrooms, thinly sliced (use an egg slicer for speed)
1 teaspoon NoSalt
½ cup grated reduced-fat Parmesan cheese
⅓ cup of sherry (optional)
Olive oil spray (optional)
Add garlic to taste

Preheat oven to 400 degrees. Place chicken breasts in pan with boiling water to cover. Add NoSalt and simmer covered for 15 to 20 minutes (checking often). Allow the chicken to rest in the broth while preparing the sauce.

Sauté mushrooms in fat-free chicken broth for five minutes. Cook garlic and mushrooms in one to two tablespoons of fat-free chicken broth or olive oil spray. Blend in remainder of broth, evaporated condensed skim milk, and sherry (if adding), stirring constantly over low heat until the sauce is smooth and thickens slightly.

Spray bottom of baking pan and layer it with chicken breast, then cover with a layer of cream sauce, reduced-fat Parmesan cheese, and mushrooms. Bake in oven until cheese is bubbling, 10 to 15 minutes. Serve with tossed salad, shredded carrots and mock mashed potatoes (see Baked Italian Cauliflower recipe).

TURKEY MARSALA

Minutes to Prepare: 10 • Minutes to Cook: 20 to 30 • Serves: 4

4 4- to 6-oz.boneless, skinless turkey breasts, sliced (pounded to a ¼-inch thickness)
Minimal flour (optional)
¼ cup low-fat, low-sodium chicken broth
¼ cup Marsala wine
¼ cup chopped fresh parsley
½ tablespoon extra virgin olive oil
NoSalt and pepper to taste
8 oz. cremini mushrooms (stems trimmed)

Season each breast with a pinch of NoSalt and pepper. Place the flour in a shallow bowl, add the turkey, and coat the pieces evenly, shaking off any excess flour.

Heat olive oil on medium in a large nonstick pan or cast iron skillet. Add the turkey, but don't overcrowd the pan (do two batches if necessary), and cook for three to four minutes a side until the breasts are golden brown on the outside and cooked all the way through. Transfer them to a serving platter and keep warm.

Add more oil to the pan, then sauté mushrooms until well browned.

Stir in the Marsala wine and broth, scraping up any browned bits stuck to bottom of pan. Cook until the liquid has reduced to about ½ cup. Season the sauce with NoSalt and pepper and add the parsley. Pour the sauce over the chicken.

GOOD-FOR-YOU CHICKEN STEW

Minutes to Prepare: 10 • Minutes to Cook: 20 to 30 • Serves: 4

I love this Chicken Stew. Fast and easy to prepare, it helps burn body fat. It's full of lean protein, vitamins, minerals, and fiber—giving your body all of the nutrients it needs to stay healthy and fit. Serve this chicken stew with a tossed salad for more oomph. Don't be afraid to adjust it to make it your own. For instance, sometimes I make it with a marinara sauce. It makes a great next-day grab-and-go lunch when you have extra.

½ teaspoon dried rosemary, crushed
½ cup fat-free, low-sodium chicken broth
½ teaspoon NoSalt (optional)
1 15.5-oz. can Cannellini beans or any other white bean, rinsed and drained
¼ teaspoon black pepper
1 lb. skinless, boneless, chicken breasts, (cut into 1-inch pieces)
1 7-oz. bottle roasted red bell peppers, drained and cut into half-inch pieces
2 teaspoons olive oil
3½ cups torn spinach
2 teaspoons jarred minced garlic or fresh

In a bowl, combine rosemary, NoSalt, black pepper, and chicken breasts. Toss well.

Heat oil in a nonstick skillet over medium-high heat. Add chicken, sauté three minutes. Add garlic, sauté one minute.

Add broth, beans, and peppers; bring to a boil. Reduce heat and simmer 10 minutes or until chicken is done. Stir in spinach, simmer one minute. Serve.

SKILLET TURKEY STEW

Minutes to Prepare: 10 • Minutes to Cook: 15 • Serves: 4

This is a fast, easy, and lean (yet hearty) main dish that you can have on your table in minutes. Skillet Turkey Stew hits the spot and makes great use of leftovers. Serve it with a salad to complete the meal. For a change, you might want to add a drained can of garbanzo (chick peas) or white beans. Turkey is a leaner and more metabolism-boosting option than chicken, but there's no reason you couldn't use chicken or even fish if you wanted.

1 tablespoon canola or olive oil or spray
1 onion, chopped
3 cups chunked cooked turkey or chicken
1 teaspoon ground cumin
1 14-oz. can no-salt-added, stewed tomatoes
1 8-oz. can whole kernel corn, drained or peas—add your favorite
1 green bell pepper, cut into chunks
¾ cup picante sauce
½ teaspoon NoSalt

In a skillet, heat oil; add onion and cook until tender, about three minutes. Add tomatoes, breaking up large pieces with a wooden spoon.

Stir in remaining ingredients; simmer 10 minutes or until green pepper is crisp-tender.

SPICY SZECHUAN CHICKEN LETTUCE WRAPS

Minutes to Prepare: 15 • Minutes to Cook: 16 • Serves: 6

This one is from my buddy Aaron McCargo, Jr.; you may have seen him on Food Network. I helped him lighten this up for those days when you feel like eating a little cleaner. I took out the butter, reduced the oil, and swapped the turkey for chicken. To make it easy, just use McCargo's Signature Blend Seasoning (available at americanspice.com).

3 8-oz. boneless skinless chicken breasts
¼ cup shredded daikon radish
2 carrots, shredded
¼ cup bean sprouts
3 stalks (½ cup) scallions
¼ cup Szechuan sauce
1 tablespoon Chinese five-spice powder
¼ teaspoon cayenne
½ teaspoon NoSalt
¼ teaspoon freshly ground black pepper
2 tablespoons grapeseed oil, for frying
1 lemon, juiced
1 head Bibb lettuce leaves

Split boneless chicken breast in half. Pound out to ¼-inch thickness if necessary.

In a medium bowl, mix together radish, carrots, bean sprouts, and scallions. Add Szechuan sauce.

In a small bowl, mix together spices, cayenne, NoSalt, and pepper. Season chicken breasts lightly with rub. Cut the chicken into strips.

In a large skillet over high heat, heat the grapeseed oil. Once hot, sear the chicken breasts for four minutes on each side. Add butter and lemon to pan and baste the chicken for another minute. Remove chicken to a platter to cool. Once cooled, dice or shred the chicken.

Place a spoonful of the vegetable mixture and the shredded chicken onto each leaf of lettuce. Roll and serve.

BISTRO (BE LEAN) BUFFALO BURGERS WITH CARAMELIZED ONIONS

Minutes to Prepare: 5 to 10 • Minutes to Cook: 15 to 20 • Serves: 4

There is nothing like the magic of seared beef—if you're a beef lover. I stopped eating red meat for over 25 years to try to control my weight, and I must admit that it wasn't easy to go back to it. That is, until I found these buffalo burgers. Buffalo meat is just as lean as turkey and provides your body with all of the amino acids needed to keep you strong and lean. If you insist on red meat (once a week—no more), you need to look for buffalo burgers if you're serious about getting lean. I pile my buffalo burger on top of a huge mound of spinach greens and top with sautéed onions. Of course, the kids get cheese and bread, but I don't miss it. This also goes great with Lean Mean Green Beans Fabrizio-Style. I like to buy my buffalo patties at Better than a Bistro (betterthanabistro.com), but you can also find ground buffalo in many supermarkets. This is so good!

> 4 Bistro Buffalo Burger patties or 1 lb. ground buffalo
> 1 large onion, sliced
> McCargo's Signature Blend Seasoning or your favorite spice
> cooking spray
> rolls (optional)

Spray pan with cooking oil and sauté onions sprinkled with McCargo's Signature Blend Seasoning or your favorite seasoning. Form into patties and grill, broil, or fry as below. Be careful not to overcook them, as they are very lean. If you overcook, add a little water to add moisture. Top each burger with sautéed onion.

If Cooking Frozen Patties
Grilling: Adjust grill so that burger surfaces are six to eight inches from coals. This gives even heat without too much intensity. If food gets too hot, raise grill away from heat.
Broiling: Preheat broiler. Top surface of burger should be 3 inches from heat. Rare: 8 minutes. Medium: 12 minutes. Well done: 20 minutes.
Frying: Preheat a heavy frying pan. When the pan is very hot, brown burgers quickly on both sides. Do not cover pan. Lower heat and cook slowly until done. Turn a few times during cooking to desired doneness.

FISH AND SEAFOOD

The lighter and whiter the fish, the better for your metabolism. Fish is good for weight loss because it's low in calories and fat and high in nutrients; it's also the best source of omega-3 fats. Simply put, the more fish you eat, the faster and easier it will be to lose weight. Frankly, I like it because you get a bigger serving. You may have seen me talk about fish on TV, and eating more seafood is the best kept diet secret on the planet. I've taken special care to create recipes that even the fussiest teens will try. Set a goal to at least find one type of seafood you'll eat, and focus on that. Also consider buying flash-frozen fish. It's more economical, and you'll never run out of healthy food as long as your freezer is stocked with flash-frozen seafood. I don't even bother with fresh anymore; instead, I rely on Vital Choice (vitalchoice.com) to deliver seafood to my doorstep.

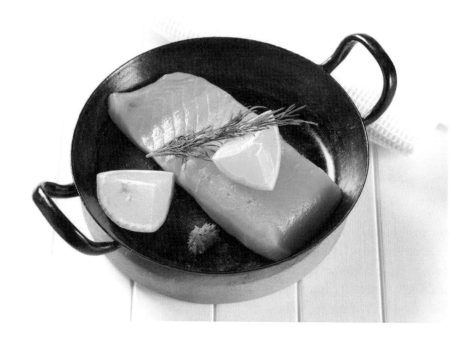

SEXY SLIMMING SALMON

Minutes to Prepare: 5 • Minutes to Cook: 10 • Number of Servings: 4

This recipe is one of the best when you're trying to cut calories because it's high in omega-3 and therefore takes a little longer to digest, which helps keep you full longer. This recipe is comforting in the winter but also grills quickly in foil. It goes great on top of a bed of spinach or baby greens along with string beans.

    4 6-oz. Alaskan salmon fillets
    4 lemon wedges
    1 tablespoon garlic powder
    1 tablespoon dried basil
    ½ teaspoon NoSalt
    1 teaspoon sesame oil

Stir together the garlic powder, basil, and NoSalt in a small bowl; rub in equal amounts onto the salmon fillets. Spray skillet with olive oil spray and place over medium heat; cook the salmon in the sesame oil until browned and flaky, about five minutes per side. Serve each piece of salmon with a lemon wedge.

ITALIAN BAKED HALIBUT
(HALIBUT A LA SICILIANO)

Minutes to Prepare: 20 • Minutes to Cook: 20 • Number of Servings: 4

My family flips for this recipe—even the picky 13-year-old fish hater. It is incredibly delicious and not too hard to make. We like this dish paired with green beans and a salad or with ciambotta.

2 pounds of Pacific halibut (may substitute tilapia, barramundi, or any other white fish)
1 large onion, sliced
1 can chopped, no-salt-added, stewed tomatoes
1 tablespoon dried basil (or 2 tablespoons fresh)
1 tablespoon dried parsley (or 2 tablespoons fresh)
1 clove of garlic, crushed
NoSalt and pepper
Sliced black olives for garnish (optional)
Dash of clam juice (red or white)

Preheat oven to 450 degrees (375 degrees for lighter fish). Wash fillets and dry with paper towels. Arrange in a single layer in 13x9 baking dish. Season with NoSalt and pepper. Cover with onions, tomatoes, basil, parsley and garlic.

Moisten with a little bit of water or clam juice. Bake for 20 minutes or just until the fish separates easily when touched with a fork. Drain off most of the liquid before serving. Garnish with black olives.

SLIMMING SEAFOOD STEW AKA CIOPPINO

Minutes to Prepare: 10 • Minutes to Cook: 30 • Number of Servings: 4

1 medium onion, quartered
1 small lemon, sliced thin
1 cup white onion, chopped
1 cup chopped red pepper
1 teaspoon oregano
1 teaspoon basil
2 bay leaves
1 tablespoon chopped parsley
3 garlic cloves, minced and/or peeled
1 tablespoon extra virgin olive oil
⅛ teaspoon dried hot red pepper flakes
1 28-oz. can crushed, no-salt-added tomatoes
1½ cups water
1 lb. of shrimp, cleaned
1 lb. cultivated mussels and/or clams
1 8-oz. bottle clam juice (optional)
1 cup balsamic vinegar or full-bodied red
1 lb. skinless fillets of thick white fish (halibut, hake, or Pollack, cut into 2-inch chunks)
wine such as Zinfandel or Syrah
1½ pounds of lobster tail, cut up into 2-inch chunks (optional)
NoSalt/pepper to taste

Chop green onion and garlic by hand or in food processor until coarse. Heat oil in a five- to six-quart heavy pot over medium-high heat and stir in quartered onion, red pepper, bay leaves, basil, oregano, red pepper flakes, NoSalt and pepper.

Cook covered over medium heat, stirring once or twice until vegetables begin to soften, about four minutes. Add tomatoes with their juice, water, balsamic vinegar or wine, clam juice (if used), lemon, and parsley; boil, covered, for 20 minutes. Stir in seafood and cook, uncovered, until fish is just cooked through and mussels open wide, approximately four to six minutes (discard any that remain unopened after six minutes). Discard bay leaves. Serve in bowls.

GAMBERI AL FORNO
(BAKED SHRIMP)

Minutes to Prepare: 5 • Minutes to Cook: 20 • Number of Servings: 2

Everyone loves shrimp—even fish haters. I love this dish for its simplicity and the sheer satisfaction I get from it. I prepare this at least once a week, especially when I have company. Pressed for time? Buy the shrimp already cleaned and cooked and sprinkle McCargo's Signature Blend Seasoning (available at americanspice.com) for a bold, delicious flavor everyone will rave about. Keep a stash of flash-frozen shrimp in your freezer so you're never without fast, easy, and healthy meal options that won't break your diet. What's the best shrimp to buy? Look for domestic shrimp; pink Oregon is my favorite. In the winter, this dish can be made in the oven; in the summer, try it on the grill in tinfoil.

14 jumbo or 20 medium shrimp
Juice of ½ lemon or 2 tablespoons of bottled lemon juice
2 to 3 cloves of garlic, chopped
Olive oil spray
Dash of paprika
⅛ cup of white wine (optional)
NoSalt and pepper (optional)

Preheat oven to 400 degrees. Peel and devein shrimp; place in a shallow baking dish sprayed with olive oil spray.

Sprinkle lemon juice and garlic over top of shrimp and spray with olive oil spray. Bake for 20 minutes or until cooked.

Add water or white wine to keep moist. Do not overcook. Check frequently. Garnish with paprika on top and NoSalt/pepper if desired.

SCALLOPS PRIMAVERA

Minutes to Prepare: 10 • Minutes to Cook: 20 • Number of Servings: 4 to 5

1 garlic clove minced
3 tomatoes, peeled and chopped
½ cup water
2 tablespoon fresh basil (or 1 tablespoon crushed, dried)
½ cup julienned carrots
1 cup broccoli florets
1 cup sliced mushrooms
1 pound of scallops (fresh or flash frozen)
1 lb. fresh asparagus
15.5-oz. can crushed, no-salt-added
1 tablespoon fresh parsley (or dried) tomatoes with basil, oregano, and onion
Reduced-fat Parmesan cheese (optional)
1 medium red bell pepper, sliced
Dash of pepper

Spray pan or wok with olive oil spray. Add garlic and cook for one minute (add some water if needed—do not let it burn).

Add water, tomato paste, carrots, broccoli, peppers and scallops if using frozen; cook for one minute.

Add scallops now if using fresh, mushrooms, tomatoes, basil, parsley, and asparagus; continue cooking until done. Pour over bed of spinach and serve immediately. Garnish with reduced-fat Parmesan cheese if desired.

SLIM-QUICK TUNA BURGERS

Minutes to Prepare: 10 • Minutes to Cook: 20 • Number of Servings: 4

Even the fish haters love these burgers. They are fast and easy to prepare and make losing weight tasty. I always suggest that you have canned tuna, salmon, or crab on hand at all times so when you run out of ideas, you always have a delicious—and good for your metabolism—backup available. You can make these burgers with ground turkey or fresh fish that you grind yourself. Of course, this recipe is leaner than most: no oil, mayonnaise, or egg yolks. Serve it on top of salad greens with green French fries (see Lean Mean Green Beans Fabrizio-Style).

2 5- to 6- oz. cans chunk light tuna in water (drained)
¼ cup finely chopped onion
¼ cup chopped celery
½ cup medium salsa
Spray oil—either olive or canola
1 egg white

Combine tuna, ¼ cup salsa, celery, and onion in a medium bowl, breaking up any larger pieces of tuna until mixture is uniform and holds together.

Combine remaining ¼ cup of salsa and egg white to tuna mixture. Spray large nonstick skillet and place over medium heat.

Using a generous ⅓ cup each, form tuna mixture into four two-inch burgers. Cook until heated through and golden brown, about two minutes per side.

Place on top of green salad and dress with your favorite salsa or mustard dressing for a big bang. Too moist? Drain excess liquid. Too dry? Add more water or salsa. Make extra for lunch during the week or for a lean snack.

CRAB CAKES GET LEAN

Minutes to Prepare: 5 • Minutes to Cook: 5 to 8 • Number of Servings: 4

1 lb. lump crabmeat, drained, shell pieces removed or 2 to 3 6-oz. cans
⅓ cup finely chopped red bell pepper
⅓ cup finely chopped green bell pepper
¼ cup light mayo or mild mustard for a leaner
1 teaspoon garlic powder version
¼ teaspoon paprika
1 teaspoon prepared mustard
3 large egg whites
2 teaspoons Worcestershire sauce or horseradish for optional zing
4 lemon wedges
Cooking spray

Preheat oven to broil. Combine everything but the lemon wedges and cooking spray in a medium bowl. Divide mixture into four equal portions, shaping each into one-inch thick patties.

Place patties on baking dish coated with cooking spray. Broil three inches from heat for eight to ten minutes or until browned. Serve with lemon wedges over a bed of baby greens.

Keep your eye on these burgers as they are very lean and cook quickly. Grill them in foil on the grill to keep moist and together. If needed, you can add a tiny bit of breadcrumbs to tighten up the patties, but I like mine as clean as possible to leave room for dessert.

GLAZED TUNA STEAKS WITH CRUNCHY CABBAGE

Minutes to Prepare: 7 • Minutes to Cook: 10 to 12 • Number of Servings: 4

Yum. And so easy to make. Great hot or cold and even better the next day. I crave this one to the point that I am always sneaking into the refrigerator to grab a bite. Thank God it's good for you. Tuna is high in omega-3, vitamin D, and selenium—all of which are necessary for your body to burn stored fat.

6 cups shredded Savoy (or any) cabbage
1 teaspoon garlic, minced
1 cup shredded purple cabbage (Timesaving tip: buy pre-shredded from a salad bar)
1 teaspoon mirin (optional; helps erase fishy smell; may also use rice wine for cooking)
2 tablespoons low-sodium soy sauce or balsamic vinegar
2 3- to 4-oz. tuna steaks (prepackaged from store are fine)
Sesame seeds (optional)
¼ cup water

Combine water, one tablespoon of the soy sauce or balsamic vinegar, mirin or rice cooking wine, and garlic in a small saucepan. Bring to a boil over medium-high heat. Stir remaining tablespoon of soy sauce into saucepan. Cook for three minutes over medium heat. Divide sauce into two separate bowls.

Place tuna in a skillet coated with cooking spray or a Teflon frying pan and add a little water so the tuna stays moist and doesn't burn. Cook/poach tuna for two to three minutes per side, depending on thickness. Drain any remaining water.

Pour half of the sauce in the saucepan; add cabbage and sauté for a few minutes until desired tenderness is reached.

Meanwhile, place cooked tuna in sprayed pan with the remaining sauce. Lightly pan sear for a minute.

Serve tuna atop a bed of the cooked cabbage.

MOJITO-GRILLED FISH TACO

Minutes to Prepare: 5 • Minutes to Cook: 14 • Number of Servings: 4

2 tablespoons lime juice
2 tablespoons mint leaves
1 whole jalapeño chili pepper, seeded and minced
½ teaspoon NoSalt (optional)
1 pound firm white fish such as halibut, red snapper, tilapia, scrod, cod, haddock, or shrimp
1 teaspoon canola oil or canola oil spray

Combine first four ingredients; stir well. Add fish to marinade. Refrigerate 20 to 30 minutes while making the rest of the meal, turning once. Remove fish from marinade and discard marinade.

Prepare grill for high-heat cooking. Place fish directly over heat; grill until firm, opaque, and lightly browned. I wrap mine in foil to keep it moist.

Not in the mood to grill? That's okay. Bake it in the oven at 350 degrees for 10-12 minutes. Cooking time may vary depending on fish and oven; keep an eye on it.

VEGETABLES

All of these recipes include fibrous, thermogenic veggies that serve as a great base for fat-free sauces (marinara) and proteins instead of pasta or starchy vegetables. My goal is to get you addicted to your own cooking to save you time and money and to help you lose that pound a day.

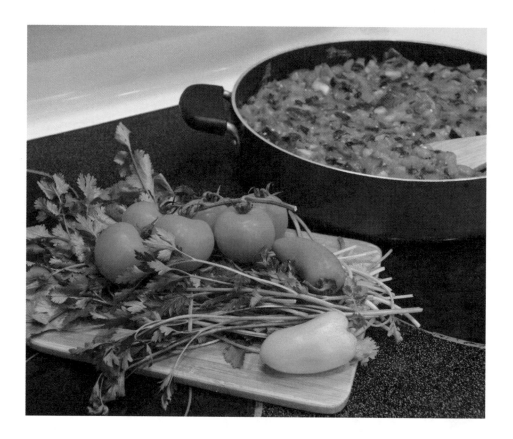

POPPA VINNIE'S CIAMBOTTA

Minutes to Prepare: 15 • Minutes to Cook: 20 • Number of Servings: 4

My grandfather used to make this hearty vegetable stew, and it is one of my all-time favorite comfort foods. It evokes such wonderful, unforgettable childhood memories for me.

1 large red bell pepper
1 large green pepper
1 32-oz. can of stewed, no-salt-added tomatoes with garlic, basil, and oregano
1 medium zucchini
1 10-oz. package mushrooms
1 medium eggplant
1 large onion
Handful of fresh basil leaves
3 minced garlic cloves
1 teaspoon olive oil
NoSalt and pepper to taste

Cut all vegetables into ¼ inch pieces. Lightly NoSalt eggplant pieces to draw out moisture and collapse their spongy texture. (It also keeps them from absorbing all the oil). Heat oil in a large skillet. Add onions, cooking until soft, then add both red and green peppers. Cook about 10 minutes on low heat. Add tomatoes, eggplant, zucchini, mushrooms, garlic, and basil. NoSalt and pepper to taste. Cook until all vegetables are soft, about 15 minutes.

BROCCOLI A LA PIZZIOLA
(BROCCOLI SICILIAN STYLE)

Minutes to Prepare: 10 • Minutes to Cook: 20 • Number of Servings: 4

This is one of my personal favorites and, quite frankly, I could live on this every day of my life. The recipe says this serves four, but I can eat the whole thing. Thank goodness more vegetables are always better when it comes to losing weight. To make a meal of it, I simply add shrimp, fish, or shredded chicken.

1 large bunch of broccoli
4 anchovy fillets, cut into pieces
1 32-oz. can chopped, no-salt-added tomatoes with basil, oregano, and garlic
1 large onion, sliced
1 tablespoon chopped garlic or garlic powder to taste
½ teaspoon pepper
½ teaspoon NoSalt
Olive oil spray (or you can use defatted or fat-free chicken broth water for steaming)
1 tablespoon grated Provolone cheese (optional)

Clean broccoli and cut into bite-size pieces. Spray bottom of pan with olive oil and place chopped onion, garlic, and one layer of broccoli in pan. Add a sprinkle of cheese, NoSalt, and pepper, then spray with olive oil until lightly covered.

Repeat layers until all broccoli is used. Spray again with olive oil and add canned tomatoes. Cover pan and cook over low heat for 15 to 20 minutes until broccoli is tender.

BAKED ITALIAN CAULIFLOWER
(METABOLIC-BOOSTING MOCK MASHED POTATOES)

Minutes to Prepare: 10 • Minutes to Cook: 20 • Number of Servings: 6

We always called this one Grandma Matasko's Baked Italian Cauliflower, and it is one of the best-tasting vegetables you'll ever eat. Every kid who comes to my house eats this up and always asks for more—despite the fact that their parents swear their kids won't eat vegetables.

    1 large head cauliflower
    olive oil spray
    ½ cup grated reduced-fat Parmesan cheese
    1 teaspoon garlic powder
    NoSalt and pepper
    1 tablespoon breadcrumbs (optional for top)

Wash and clean cauliflower; break into florets. Boil for five minutes in NoSalted water until half cooked. Drain. You can also microwave it or steam it on the stovetop instead of boiling.

Spray bottom of baking dish with olive oil spray and arrange cauliflower on bottom. Combine bread-crumbs (if used) with grated reduced-fat Parmesan cheese and sprinkle over cauliflower. Season with pepper and garlic powder. Spray top to coat with olive oil spray.

Bake at 350 degrees for 15 to 20 minutes. If it becomes dry, add water to keep moist. Cooking times may vary depending on oven; keep in mind you're cooking very lean which means little or no oils and fat, so things cook faster and dry out quicker, making it necessary sometimes to add liquid to the dish.

LEAN MEAN GREEN BEANS FABRIZIO-STYLE

Minutes to Prepare: 5 • Minutes to Cook: 5 to 10 • Number of Servings: 4 to 6

Every person I have ever worked with who hates vegetables loves green beans. My 13-year-old fussy eater calls these green French fries. They are a great finger food—even delicious cold. I make these green beans every single week to guarantee my kids eat their vegetables without my asking. Even with ketchup, they're still healthier than French fries. They also serve as a great grab-and-go snack. Just store them in a plastic container so they're ready to go when you are.

> 1 lb. fresh green beans (or whole frozen green beans)
> 1 32-oz. can chopped, no-salt-added tomatoes with garlic, basil, and oregano
> 1 to 2 tablespoons chopped garlic (jarred works)
> NoSalt and pepper
> Olive oil spray

If preparing fresh beans, cut off tips, remove any strings and break in half. Cook quickly in undrained chopped tomatoes until crisp-tender (do not overcook). Keep cover off to retain vibrant green color. Cool to room temperature under running water as soon as you remove from heat to stop further cooking.

If preparing frozen, follow package instructions for cooking beans. Or simply thaw if making cold.

Place cooked beans in serving bowl. Spray with olive oil and season with garlic, NoSalt, and pepper.

PASTA NOT!—CARROTS, ZUCCHINI, & SQUASH RIBBONS

Minutes to Prepare: 10 • Minutes to Cook: 10 • Number of Servings: 6

Do you ever wonder how you'll survive without pasta? I used to ask myself that question. What I've learned is that it wasn't the pasta I was addicted to, but rather the sauces. Pasta is nothing more than a fattening, metabolic-slowing food that is highly overrated. I substitute Pasta Not! for pasta under my turkey meatballs with sauce. And you can have plenty of Pasta Not! because it's practically calorie-free. If you're craving a big bowl of buttery noodles, trick yourself by eating yellow squash with your favorite seasoning. Never use butter unless you want to gain weight. The more Pasta Not! you eat, the leaner you'll be.

    3 large yellow squash, peeled
    3 large zucchini, peeled
    2 large carrots
    2 tablespoons fat-free chicken stock
    2 to 3 teaspoons minced or chopped garlic (jarred is fine)
    ¼ teaspoon black pepper
    ½ teaspoon NoSalt (optional)
    Juice from ½ lime or 2 tablespoons bottled lime juice (optional)

Cut or slice squash, carrots and zucchini into thin ribbons with a mandoline slicer or, as we Italians do it, by hand with a knife.

In a large skillet, heat chicken stock over medium heat. Add garlic and cook for two minutes, adding more stock or water if it dries out too quickly.

Add carrot ribbons. Toss in zucchini and squash ribbons, NoSalt and pepper. Cook for 5 to 10 minutes. Keep an eye on it because it is fat-free and may cook quickly and/or dry out. Season with lime juice if desired.

ROASTED ASPARAGUS BUNDLES

Minutes to Prepare: 5 • Minutes to Cook: 25 • Number of Servings: 4

Asparagus is full of vitamins K, A, and C as well as iron, thiamin, folate, and fiber. It's a good choice for when you need an easy, go-to vegetable—or when you want to feel less bloated. Did you know that asparagus is a natural diuretic? Fitness pros and models eat asparagus the day before a shoot to help rid the body of excess water. I love to eat these bundles with fish or on top of a salad. And they're great cold the next day as a finger food when I need to munch. Serve with any lean protein.

> 1 lb. fresh asparagus spears, tough ends trimmed and discarded (about 5 to 6
>   stalks per serving)
> ½ teaspoon NoSalt
> Olive oil cooking spray or 1 tablespoon or less of extra virgin olive oil

Preheat oven to 400 degrees. Place asparagus on a baking sheet. Spray with olive oil cooking spray or drizzle with olive oil and sprinkle with NoSalt. Roast 25 to 30 minutes, until tender.

Wrap individual portions of asparagus with asparagus to tie into bundles.

LISA LYNN'S HEALTH-BOOSTING CARROT OVEN FRIES

Minutes to Prepare: 5 • Minutes to Cook: 25 • Number of Servings: 4 to 6

This is my secret way of getting kids who visit my house to eat their veggies. And guess what I have learned in the 25 years of helping people lose weight? There are many grownups who hate veggies too. While the Hidden Valley Ranch seasoning isn't perfect, it does give added flavor and serves as a little motivation to do the right thing: eat vegetables. These carrots are simple and inexpensive to make, which is a good thing because you will never have any leftovers. These go great with turkey or tuna burgers to keep the meal healthy and balanced but still fun.

1 lb. carrots (about 5 or 6 large, peeled and cut in 4 ¼-inch sticks) or a 1 lb. bag of
   baby carrots
1 packet Hidden Valley Original Ranch Dressing and Seasoning mix
Vegetable cooking spray

Preheat oven to 400 degrees. In a large bowl, combine carrots with olive oil and half the packet of dry Hidden Valley Original Ranch Salad Dressing Seasoning Mix. Toss until well coated.

Spray pan generously with cooking spray. Arrange carrots in a single layer on pan and bake 25 to 30 minutes or until crispy.

AUNT HEDWIG'S CABBAGE AND ONIONS TO DIE FOR

Minutes to Prepare: 10 • Minutes to Cook: 20 to 30 • Number of Servings: 6 to 8

Who knew a simple cabbage recipe could be so delicious? Cabbage is a nutritional powerhouse, but what most people don't know is that you practically burn more calories eating this vegetable than digesting it. It is a great thermogenic food that revs up your metabolism. My Polish Aunt Hedwig made this recipe and, no matter the age, everyone in the family licked their plates clean. My Grandpa Vinnie liked to add a can of crushed no-salt-added tomatoes to the cabbage while cooking. Feel free to get creative by adding turkey or chicken—whatever your family likes.

1 large head of cabbage (I like Savoy best)
2 medium onions
1 tablespoon of your favorite vinegar such as cider, white wine, or sherry
2 to 3 tbsp. fat-free chicken broth
1 teaspoon olive oil
1 teaspoon caraway, cumin, fenugreek, or fennel
NoSalt and freshly ground pepper
1 32-oz. can crushed, no-salt-added tomatoes (optional)
1 clove minced garlic (optional)
Black pepper to taste (optional)

Quarter the cabbage and cut out the core. Slice the cabbage as thinly as possible and set it aside. (You can use a food processor or kitchen mandoline, if you like, or cut it by hand.) Halve, peel, and slice the onions as thinly as possible.

Heat a large pot or deep sauté pan over medium-high heat. Add the oil and chicken broth. When hot, add the onions, sprinkling them with NoSalt, and cook until the onions wilt, about three minutes. Add the cabbage and garlic (if using), sprinkling with NoSalt again, and stir to combine. Reduce heat to low and cook, covered, until the vegetables are extremely tender, about 20 to 30 minutes, stirring occasionally. If using, add caraway, cumin, fenugreek, or fennel at this point. Add crushed tomatoes if desired to turn this dish into a yummy cabbage stew. Add one or two tablespoons of water to keep vegetables from sticking if necessary.

MUSHROOMS AND SPINACH ITALIAN STYLE

Minutes to Prepare: 10 • Minutes to Cook: 10 • Number of Servings: 4

4 tablespoons fat-free chicken broth
Olive oil spray
1 small onion, chopped
2 cloves of garlic, chopped
14 oz. fresh mushrooms (I adore baby bellas)
1 tablespoon of balsamic vinegar
10 oz. clean fresh spinach, (chop if desired)
NoSalt and pepper to taste

Spray a large skillet and heat fat-free chicken broth over medium-high heat. Sauté onion and garlic until they start to become tender.

Add mushrooms and sauté until they begin to shrink, about three to four minutes.

Toss in the spinach, stirring constantly until spinach is wilted.

Add the balsamic vinegar, reduce heat to low, and simmer until the liquid is almost completely absorbed. Season with NoSalt and pepper to taste.

FAT-MELTING ONIONS AND PEPPER

Minutes to Prepare: 10 • Minutes to Cook: 10 • Number of Servings: 4

Everyone needs to know how to make killer onions and peppers. My Aunt Angie showed me this. These veggies not only turn up the dial on your metabolism but they are delicious hot or cold. I love the smell permeating the house when I'm preparing this dish, and I adore it when my kids walk in and say, "Yummm! What's for dinner?" and start grabbing at these veggies.

1 medium-sized red pepper
1 medium-sized yellow pepper
1 medium yellow onion
1 medium-sized green pepper
1 medium-sized orange pepper
2 tablespoons red wine vinegar
NoSalt and pepper (optional)
2 cloves garlic, finely minced (optional)
Olive oil spray

Start chopping. Cut your onions in half, then quarters. Chop the onions in such a way that you end up with half circle strips. Slice peppers into long strips about ⅛ of an inch thick. Chop garlic into smallest mince possible.

Spray medium skillet with olive oil spray and heat on medium. Be sure spray covers every part of the pan.

Cook sliced onions and peppers in the skillet for 10 minutes, stirring occasionally. Turn heat to low after 10 minutes to keep onions from burning and to allow them to soften. Add garlic when you turn down the heat. Want more spice? Add a pinch of NoSalt and pepper for flavor. Stir in the red wine vinegar, and you're ready to eat.

ZUCCHINI-INTO-YOUR-BIKINI PARMESAN CRISPS

Minutes to Prepare: 15   •   Minutes to Cook: 30   •   Number of Servings: 4

This is how you break the potato chip habit. Why grab crispy chips and blow your diet when you can eat these? I make these at least once a week. What makes this recipe extra lean? No egg yolk and very, very little oil.

2 medium zucchini (about 1 pound total)
¼ cup freshly grated reduced-fat Parmesan cheese
Approximately ¼ cup Italian bread crumbs
Cooking spray

Preheat the oven to 450 degrees. Coat baking sheet with cooking spray. (You can also cook these in a toaster oven where they heat up fast and get crispy even faster.)

Slice zucchini into ¼-inch-thick rounds. Spray a medium bowl with cooking spray and toss the zucchini to coat.

In a small bowl combine the reduced-fat Parmesan and breadcrumbs. Dip each round into the Parmesan mixture, coating it evenly on both sides, pressing the coating on to stick, and place in a single layer on the prepared baking sheet.

Bake the zucchini rounds until browned and crisp, 25 to 30 minutes. Remove with spatula. Serve immediately.

PORTOBELLO UN-PIZZA

Minutes to Prepare: 5 • Minutes to Cook: 12 • Number of Servings: 1

When I was little, I was a chubette. Here's an embarrassing confession: All my relatives used to call me Lisa Pizza—and I didn't get that name for nothin'. I craved pizza and could never get enough. My pizza craving didn't go away as I grew older, either. I could never stop at one slice, and then I could never work it off in the gym. I finally found a lean solution: While my family eats pizza, I eat a guilt-free Portobello UN-Pizza. Get creative. You'll never miss the cheese if you add shrimp or turkey meatballs, and your flatter stomach will show up sooner. Make it thermogenic by adding three ounces of precooked chicken breast. These pizzas can also be made on squash slices for an even lighter meal that fills you up, not out. And guess what? My family now fights over these.

    1 Portobello mushroom, 4 to 5 inches in diameter
    Olive oil spray
    3 tablespoons marinara or other tomato-based sauce (look for low-fat, no sugar added)
    NoSalt and black pepper to taste
    1 teaspoon reduced-fat Parmesan, grated (optional)

Preheat oven to 425 degrees. If mushroom has a stem, slice it off close to the cap (reserve for soups or sauces). Spray cap with olive oil and place stem side up on a rimmed baking sheet or pan. Sprinkle lightly with NoSalt and pepper. Bake 15 minutes until mushroom is hot. Spread sauce on cap and top with cheese if using.

KALE CHIPS

Minutes to Prepare: 5 • Minutes to Cook: 30 • Number of Servings: Why measure?

Kale is big on the health food radar these days. Truth is, I don't love kale, but I do love to munch and crunch during anxious times so this is just what I need. An awesome client who has lost 60 pounds turned me on to this recipe. It's a great potato chip replacement and so easy your kids can make these. If you want to cut down on the oil, use a spray—you won't have to use a bag then either. Be creative and use your favorite spices. And try substituting with string beans or whatever veggies you have in the house. Just remember to adjust the cooking time.

Big bunch of kale greens
1 tablespoon olive oil or cooking spray
1 teaspoon balsamic vinegar
Large zip-top bag
Salt-free Mrs. Dash (optional) or NoSalt

Wash kale greens and dry thoroughly with paper towels. Tear off two-inch portions of the leaves. Discard stems as they are bitter. Place the leaves in zip-top bag. Add olive oil and balsamic vinegar. Close bag and "massage" to distribute evenly over the kale leaves. (The bag keeps your fingers from getting messy.)

Remove leaves and place in single layer onto cookie sheet lined with parchment paper. Sprinkle with NoSalt or Mrs. Dash. Roast in oven at 350 degrees for 30 minutes.

THE INCREDIBLE METABOLIC-BOOSTING EGG WHITE

If you're trying to boost your metabolism so you can finally lose weight, and you hate fish, egg whites are your new best friend. They are one of the best sources of protein and have no fat. Not just for breakfast anymore, egg whites make some of the best quick delicious meals. Armed with these delicious and filling recipes, you will never have an excuse to not eat lean and clean. And don't forget about the basic hard-boiled egg—just discard the yolk. Did you know that one yolk has 7 grams of fat? That's almost half of your daily fat allowance of 15 to 20 grams when trying to lose weight. And don't buy into the ads claiming that yolks contain "good" fat. If you're out to lose weight, you have to reduce your fat intake, no ifs, ands, or buts about it. Keep a stash of hard-boiled egg whites in your refrigerator for those moments when you need to pop something into your mouth.

POMODORINI CON UOVE DI FABRIZIO

Minutes to Prepare: 5 • Minutes to Cook: 10 • Number of Servings: 2

My grandfather used to make this dish for me with his ciambotto. It makes egg whites seem like a special treat.

1 medium onion, sliced
½ can crushed, peeled, no-salt-added tomatoes
Chopped parsley (optional)
Olive or canola oil spray
8 egg whites
NoSalt and pepper (optional)

Spray a small frying pan with olive or canola oil; spray and sauté onions until wilted and soft. Add a little water if too dry. Add tomatoes and parsley (if using) and cook for 5 to 10 minutes, stirring often.

As tomatoes simmer, gently break eight eggs, separating the white and discarding the yolk. Poach whites in boiling water until cooked to your liking. Add a salad on the side or any leftover vegetables directly to the eggs, and you've got a delicious metabolism-boosting meal that's done in 10 minutes.

EGG WHITE BITES

Minutes to Prepare: 10 • Minutes to Cook: 6 to 8 • Number of Servings: 6

I always have these in my refrigerator; they are great to pop into your mouth when you just gotta munch. Your whole family will love them and be eating healthier with these Egg White Bites. They pack great in kids' lunch boxes and in yours too. Top salads with them or have them as a lean snack to help reach your protein quota. My son Kyle loves to make these, and that gets him to eat them, too. Mothers of wrestlers: This will get a big smile as it will help your son stay healthy and make his weight class. Egg White Bites make a great post-workout snack, refueling your muscles.

2 cups Egg Beater egg whites or 12 egg whites
Cooking spray
2 plum tomatoes, chopped, seeded, and drained
1 teaspoon chopped basil (optional)
1 teaspoon chopped garlic (optional)
NoSalt and pepper to taste

Preheat oven to 350 degrees. Spray a nonstick muffin tin with cooking spray. Drop one egg white or the Egg Beater equivalent into each well of the muffin tin. Place one teaspoon of chopped tomato on each egg white and sprinkle with NoSalt and pepper if desired. Garnish with chopped basil.

Place on center oven rack and bake for six to eight minutes or until egg whites reach desired doneness.

Get creative. Add any vegetable to the Egg White Bite. Spinach, asparagus, broccoli, peppers, onions, an oriental blend—all are great. Add salsa, hot sauce, or your favorite spice.

SALMON AND ASPARAGUS FRITTATA

Minutes to Prepare: 10 • Minutes to Cook: 20 • Number of Servings: 4

My husband doesn't cook much, so it's a treat when he does. This is Jeff's specialty. We all look forward to Sunday brunch and hope there will be leftovers for lunch on Monday. This frittata makes an awesome lunch or dinner, too. For a salmon touch that will absolutely dazzle you, try Vital Choice's salmon bacon (vitalchoice.com). It's perfect for that extra special meal.

> 12 egg whites (lightly beaten)
> NoSalt and pepper (optional)
> Olive oil spray
> 1 cup chopped onion
> ½ cup red bell pepper, diced
> 1 8-oz. salmon fillet, skin removed and cut into bite-size pieces
> ½ teaspoon oregano

Preheat broiler. Combine egg whites with NoSalt and pepper (if using) in a bowl.

Spray large ovenproof skillet with cooking spray. Over medium-high heat, cook onion, bell pepper, and oregano, stirring occasionally until vegetables are somewhat soft, about three minutes.

Add asparagus and cook three minutes. Add salmon and cook until opaque, approximately three minutes.

Pour egg mixture into skillet and reduce heat to low, stirring occasionally until eggs begin to set but are still wet on top, about five minutes. Cook for an additional five minutes without stirring. Transfer skillet to broiler and broil until golden, two to three minutes. Serve with salad.

THE HEARTY (I'M STARVING!) OMELET

Minutes to Prepare: None • Minutes to Cook: 5 • Number of Servings: 2

At my house, this is the "I'm-starving-I-could-eat-a-horse" omelet. In those moments, we get very creative; I open the fridge and take out whatever I have available (usually ciambotta) and scramble it in a pan with three egg whites per person. Add a sprinkle of reduced-fat Parmesan cheese and you have a meal fast. Make one day a week omelet night to help you lose weight faster. You can mix in any food on the metabolic-boosting food lists. Just remember, if you don't see a food listed, don't eat it. If I don't list a food, that means it's not good for weight loss. Old food faves like bacon, cheese (even low-fat) and any kind of red meat do not boost your metabolism.

> 6 egg whites
> Spray oil
> Your favorite leftover or ingredient

Spray pan. Add three whisked egg whites. Cook until solid. Add filling, flip omelet half over to close. Cook an additional one to two minutes. Serve. Repeat with remaining egg whites and filling.

EGG WHITE FLORENTINE IN A TOMATO CUP

Minutes to Prepare: 5 • Minutes to Cook: 25 • Number of Servings: 4

8 large egg whites (separated) at room temperature, whipped
4 large beefsteak tomatoes
¼ cup minced shallots
Olive oil spray or 1 teaspoon olive oil
¼ cup low-sodium chicken broth
1 10-oz. package frozen spinach, thawed and squeezed of all excess liquid
¼ cup grated reduced-fat Parmesan cheese
NoSalt and pepper (optional)

Preheat oven to 400 degrees. Slice off top of each tomato and, using a melon baller, scoop out the insides of the tomatoes; do not discard. Make sure to leave the outside intact to form a cup. Place the hollowed out tomatoes on a foil-lined baking sheet.

Heat a medium nonstick skillet over medium heat. Spray with cooking spray, then add shallots and cook for two minutes or until shallots are translucent. Whisk in broth and cook for two to three minutes or until warm. Add spinach and tomato pulp and cook, stirring two to three minutes or until liquid is evaporated. Stir in half of the reduced-fat Parmesan cheese and NoSalt and pepper if desired (cheese has enough salt, trust me).

Fill one tomato with ⅓ cup of spinach mixture. Then form a small well in the center. Carefully pour whipped egg whites into center of the spinach well; repeat with remaining tomatoes. Sprinkle each tomato with remaining Parmesan cheese and bake for 15 to 20 minutes or until egg whites are set. Serve immediately.

Rushed? Bake the tomatoes as soon as they are hollow; cook the egg whites with the spinach mixture in the skillet. Then put the warm mixture into the heated tomato shells. If using reduced-fat Parmesan, sprinkle on top and put under broiler just long enough to melt the cheese. This method cuts the cooking time in half.

THE SALAD OMELET

Minutes to Prepare: 10 • Minutes to Cook: 5 • Number of Servings: 2

6 large egg whites or 1½ cups egg-white substitute
3 cups mixed baby greens or mesclun mix (my preference)
½ cup grape tomatoes
¼ cup roughly chopped flat-leafed parsley
1 teaspoon extra virgin olive oil or olive oil spray
1 tablespoon red wine vinegar
NoSalt and pepper to taste (optional)

Position a rack on the shelf closest to broiler and preheat broiler to high.

Toss the tomatoes with the vinegar and spray with olive oil or toss using half the teaspoon. Season with NoSalt and pepper; set aside.

Warm a medium nonstick oven-ready skillet over medium-low heat. Whisk the egg whites in a large bowl until foamy and doubled in volume. Season with NoSalt and pepper and whisk in parsley. Add the remaining olive oil to the skillet or, better yet, spray it.

Pour egg whites into the skillet and swirl to cover entire skillet. Cook, without stirring, until the whites are almost set and light brown on the bottom, about three minutes.

Set the skillet under the hot broiler and cook until the omelet sets and begins to brown, about 30 seconds. Spoon half the tomato mixture onto half the omelet, then fold the empty side over filling. Transfer omelet to a serving platter and arrange the remaining tomato salad on top. Serve with baby greens on the side. You can also stuff the omelet with the baby greens before folding over—that's my favorite.

COFFEE CUP SCRAMBLE
(THE THREE-MINUTE EGG WHITE)

Minutes to Prepare: 1 • Minutes to Cook: 2 • Number of Servings: 1

This recipe works for those hard-to-get- protein times like vacations, when at the office, or when you're going to have an extremely long day and need warm, real food. I like this recipe because my kids and husband will eat it. Breakfast is the most important meal of the day, but that doesn't mean you default to eating carbohydrates. Protein provides sustainable energy and keeps our minds sharp and our bodies ready to go. When you need a quick protein pick-me-up, try this one. You can add turkey sausage, vegetables, salmon, or your favorite spice and make it your own.

2 to 3 egg whites or equivalent amount of egg white substitute
1 teaspoon mild salsa
Spray oil

Spray to coat a 12- to 16- oz. microwave-safe coffee mug with cooking spray. Add egg whites and beat in salsa until blended. Microwave on high 45 seconds and stir, then microwave an additional 30 to 45 seconds or until cooked. Microwave cooking times may vary so adjust accordingly.

SLIMMING SOUPS

Soup is one of the best-kept secrets when it comes to losing weight. It's fast, filling and, if it's packed with the right ingredients like light broths (fat-free and low-sodium of course), vegetables, and lean proteins, it's good for your metabolism. These recipes are simple to make and so delicious you'll crave them day after day. These soups have minimal calories and are full of thermogenic vegetables that will rev up your metabolism. Soups will not only keep you feeling full, but they will help you lose weight faster. They are also a great way to keep yourself hydrated. Finally, a comfort food that's good for you!

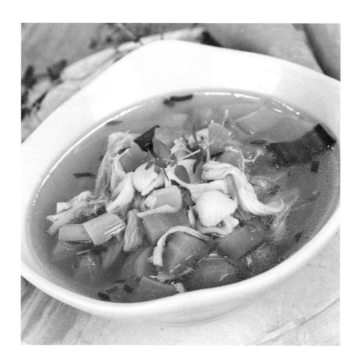

CHICKEN SOUP FOR THE METABOLISM

Minutes to Prepare: 15 • Minutes to Cook: 30 • Number of Servings: 4

8 cups chicken stock or fat-free, low-sodium chicken broth
2 4-oz. skinless, bone-in chicken thighs
1 12-oz. skinless, bone-in half chicken breast
2 cups diagonally sliced carrots
2 cups diagonally sliced celery
1 cup chopped onion
½ teaspoon NoSalt
½ teaspoon black pepper
Celery leaves (optional)

Combine the first three ingredients in a large pot over medium-high heat; bring to a boil. Reduce heat and simmer 20 minutes.

Remove chicken from pot; let stand for 10 minutes. Remove chicken from bones; shred meat into bite-size pieces. Discard bones.

Add carrots, celery, and onion to pot; cover and simmer for 10 minutes. Add chicken, NoSalt, and black pepper; cook until vegetables are tender. Garnish with celery leaves if desired.

LEMONY SPINACH SOUP

Minutes to Prepare: 15 • Minutes to Cook: 30 • Number of Servings: 4

This is one of the lightest and most refreshing soups you'll ever try. This soup can be turned into a meal by adding strips of chicken or shrimp. For a vegetarian version of this lemony soup, use organic or low-sodium vegetable broth in place of chicken broth.

- 1 teaspoon extra virgin olive oil
- 3 garlic cloves, thinly sliced
- 2 thinly sliced green onions
- 1 15-oz. can no-salt-added chickpeas (garbanzo beans), drained
- 4 cups fat-free, low-sodium chicken broth
- 2 cups water
- 1 tablespoon grated lemon rind
- 1 tablespoon chopped fresh oregano
- 1 tablespoon lemon juice
- ½ teaspoon freshly ground black pepper
- ⅛ teaspoon NoSalt
- 1 6-oz. package fresh baby spinach
- ⅓ cup grated reduced-fat Parmesan cheese (optional)

Heat a large saucepan over high heat. Add olive oil and swirl to coat. Add garlic and onions and sauté 30 seconds, stirring constantly.

Add chicken broth and two cups of water; bring to a boil. Add lemon rind and chickpeas. Cover and cook 10 minutes.

Stir in oregano, black pepper, lemon juice, NoSalt, and spinach. Ladle 1 ¾ cups of soup into each of four bowls. Top each serving with a sprinkle of reduced-fat Parmesan cheese.

GIGI'S ZUPPA DI SCAROLA
(ESCAROLE SOUP)

Minutes to Prepare: 15 • Minutes to Cook: 30 • Number of Servings: 4

Growing up, my younger brother Gary ("Gigi") was the cook in our house, and one of the things he made very well was escarole soup. It was probably the only healthy thing we ate. It is one of the easiest, most delicious soups to make. This version is a metabolic-boosting version, so the carbohydrates and fat are removed. This soup can easily be made into a meal by adding thin strips of chicken pulled off the bone or floating some shrimp in it. On a weekend as a special treat, I'll add turkey sausage.

1 head escarole, cut into bite-size pieces
2 tablespoons chopped carrots
4 cups fat-free, low-sodium chicken broth
2 cups water
NoSalt and pepper
Reduced-fat Parmesan cheese, optional

Simmer escarole, carrots, and chicken broth seasoned with NoSalt for 20 minutes. Add black pepper and water; stir well. Ladle hot soup into bowls. Sprinkle with reduced-fat Parmesan cheese if desired.

ZUPPA DI SPOSALIZIO
(ITALIAN WEDDING SOUP GONE LEAN)

Minutes to Prepare: 10 • Minutes to Cook: 15 • Number of Servings: 4

If you grew up Italian, you know we never waste one single meatball. We eat them every possible way. And since the turkey meatballs in this book are so lean, you can eat them every day. This is a very simple and fast soup you can make in 20 minutes or less and leave the table feeling satisfied without slowing your metabolism.

 4 cups fat-free chicken broth
 1 small onion, sliced into rings
 2 teaspoons NoSalt (optional)
 2 cups of water
 4 cups of romaine lettuce leaves (spinach or escarole work well also)
 Turkey meatballs (from prior recipe)

Put broth and onion in a large pot and cook over medium heat for three to five minutes until hot. Add the water and turkey meatballs, then cook two to three more minutes or until warm. Do not boil or overcook. Add romaine leaves at the end as they cook very fast. Ladle into large soup bowl and mangia! Want seconds? Go for it.

GET LEAN GAZPACHO

Minutes to Prepare: 15 • Minutes to Cook: N/A • Number of Servings: 4

Gazpacho is one of the easiest soups to make, and it's one of the healthiest. It's also super delicious. This recipe is leaner and cleaner because I don't add oil, which jacks up the calories. I also like my gazpacho chunkier, so I make it in a food processor by pulsing it until the desired thickness is reached.

2 Roma (plum) tomatoes, chopped
½ cucumber, chopped
½ green bell pepper, chopped
½ red bell pepper, chopped
½ small red onion, chopped
1 clove garlic, minced
2 cups tomato juice
2 teaspoons beef bouillon granules
½ teaspoon dried oregano
½ teaspoon dried basil
¼ teaspoon celery salt
¼ teaspoon NoSalt
⅛ teaspoon ground black pepper
1½ teaspoons Worcestershire sauce
1½ teaspoons red wine vinegar

Puree Roma tomatoes, cucumber, green and red bell peppers, red onion, and garlic in food processor or blender about 30 seconds. Add tomato juice, beef bouillon granules, oregano, basil, celery salt, NoSalt, black pepper, Worcestershire sauce, and red wine vinegar. Pulse a few times to mix. Pour into a bowl and chill at least 1 hour.

Like your gazpacho thicker? Pulse tomatoes in the food processor until desired texture is achieved. Pour into a bowl. Repeat with the bell peppers (I use red, green, and yellow) and onions, and pour into the same bowl. Repeat again with cucumbers. This allows you to control the texture of all the vegetables. Finally, add the bouillon, oregano, basil, seasonings, Worcestershire, and red wine vinegar, then pulse to mix. Add to the bowl with the other processed veggies. In a rush? Use frozen peppers or precut ones from your market salad bar.

ROMAN EGG DROP SOUP
(EGG WHITE DROP THE POUNDS SOUP)

Minutes to Prepare: 5 • Minutes to Cook: 5 • Number of Servings: 2 to 3

Egg drop soup is very popular in Rome, but it is so high in cholesterol. I make a leaner version that is good for boosting your metabolism rather than slowing it down. You'll never miss the yolks—and that's where all the fat is. Removing the yolk saves you seven grams of fat per yolk.

    4 cups chicken broth
    6 egg whites
    1 tablespoon chopped scallions
    Add your favorite vegetables (optional)

Place broth in medium-size pot and bring to slow boil. Whip/beat egg whites until thick but not stiff. Gently and slowly pour egg whites into simmering broth, stirring gently. Continue to stir and simmer for two to three minutes. Serve topped with scallions.

Need more flavor? Add ½ cup of sweet onions. Simply sauté them in a sprayed pan for one to two minutes before adding broth.

MELT FAT MINESTRONE
(ITALIAN CABBAGE SOUP)

Minutes to Prepare: 15 • Minutes to Cook: 40 • Number of Servings: 8

If you think cabbage soup is effective when it comes to weight loss, wait until you try this. The difference? You'll actually like this one. This soup is one of the staples in my house. I leave out the pasta for myself, but add it to my husband's and kids' soup bowls since they need the carbs and I don't.

Spray olive oil
1 garlic clove, chopped
¼ head of cabbage, shredded*
3 stalks of celery, diced
¼ pound of green beans, cut into 1-inch pieces
3 carrots, sliced
2 cups fat-free beef broth (vegetable soups work for vegans, too)
3 small zucchini chopped
1 6-oz. can of tomato paste
1 15-oz. can of kidney beans
1 cup of chopped onion
9 cups of water
1 tablespoon of parsley

Spray large pot with olive oil spray, then sauté onions, garlic, parsley, celery, cabbage, carrots, and green beans until wilted. Add tomato paste, beef broth, and water and simmer for twenty minutes. Add beans and zucchini and cook for five to twenty more minutes.

Serve topped with a dash of reduced-fat Parmesan cheese if desired.

*Not a cabbage eater? Substitute your favorite vegetable, like yellow squash or spinach. Need more flavor? Add a dash of hot sauce or sprinkle in your favorite seasoning, like McCargo's Signature Blend or Mrs. Dash.

VERY QUICK VEGETARIAN CHILI

Minutes to Prepare: 10   •   Minutes to Cook: 25   •   Number of Servings: 6

Finally, comfort food that is good for you! This is a great way to reduce calories after a not-so-good eating day. This recipe is practically free it's so healthy. Need protein? Add some cooked turkey chunks instead of beans to keep calories low. And when you're pressed for time, you can always use low-sodium taco seasoning (aka Turkey Joe's in my house) and add loads of veggies. I like to add green vegetables and use "steamer" frozen veggies so I don't have to spend my time chopping. Be sure to make extra and freeze it in single storage containers so it's always ready to grab and go. Enjoy.

2 teaspoons canola oil
1 cup chopped onion
1 cup chopped red bell pepper
2 teaspoons chili powder
1 teaspoon ground cumin
1 teaspoon dried oregano
3 cloves of garlic, minced
1 4.5-oz. can chopped green chilis
¼ cup water
1 15-oz. can black beans, drained
1 14.5-oz. can no-salt-added, diced tomatoes, undrained
1 14-oz. can low-sodium, vegetable broth
3 tablespoons chopped fresh cilantro
Precooked turkey chunks (optional)
6 lime wedges

Heat the oil in a large saucepan on medium-high heat. Add the onion and bell pepper; sauté until soft, about three to five minutes.

Add chili powder, cumin, oregano, garlic, and green chilis. Cook one minute. Stir in water, black beans, diced tomatoes and vegetable broth. Bring to a boil; cover; reduce heat and simmer 15 to 20 minutes. Stir in cilantro.

Serve with lime wedges.

SALADS

Salads are not just for the salad bowl. These awesome, slimming, thermogenic wonders can be sautéed if you crave warm comfort food. They work great under your favorite protein—place your favorite fish or chicken on top of a salad instead of pasta. Salads are especially great as fillers, stopping you from overindulging on a perhaps not-so-fat-free main course. Any time you want to fill up, try adding some fat-free chicken broth or your favorite bouillon over your salad for a delicious, hot, almost-calorie-free soup.

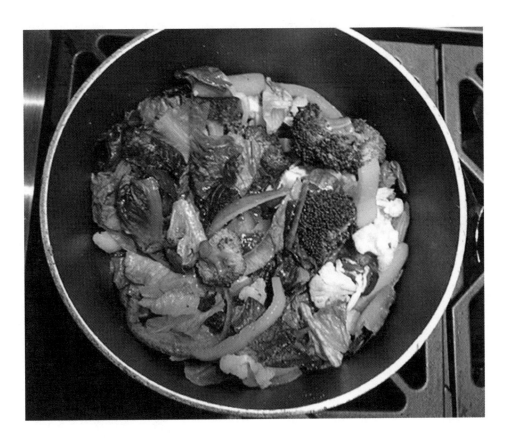

LISA'S FAMOUS SAUTÉED SALAD

Minutes to Prepare: 5 • Minutes to Cook: 10 • Number of Servings: 2

Spray olive oil or ½ tablespoon or less of extra virgin olive oil (use as little as possible)
1 small, sweet onion such as white or Vidalia, thinly sliced
3 heads romaine lettuce (substitute chopped escarole or broccoli rabe if you wish)
Choose your own vegetables to add
¼ teaspoon NoSalt
Grated reduced-fat Parmesan (optional)

Heat oil in 12-inch skillet over medium heat. Add onion and cook, stirring often, for 10 minutes or until golden. Lower heat if onion is browning too quickly; don't let it brown. Add romaine to skillet and cook, turning occasionally, for about two to three minutes, until leaves are tender yet still crunchy. Sprinkle with salt substitute. Garnish with grated cheese if desired.

CLEANEST SKINNY CAESAR SALAD

Minutes to Prepare: 10 to 15 • Number of Servings: 2

1 large garlic clove, chopped
2 teaspoons Dijon mustard
Juice of ½ lemon
4 anchovies, rinsed
4 cups chopped romaine
NoSalt and pepper
Grilled chicken or shrimp*
1 teaspoon Worcestershire
Reduced-fat Parmesan cheese
Croutons (optional)
¼ cup fat-free chicken broth or extra virgin olive oil

Combine Worcestershire, Dijon, anchovies, lemon, and garlic in blender, slowly adding the chicken broth or extra virgin olive oil. Mix with the chopped romaine and top with grilled chicken or shrimp and reduced-fat Parmesan cheese. Generously season with NoSalt and pepper.

*I marinate the chicken in nonfat Italian dressing.

LISA'S BE-HEALTHY SALAD

Minutes to Prepare: 10 to 15 • Number of Servings: 4

SIMPLE SALAD DRESSING

> 1 to 2 teaspoons red wine vinegar
> Canola oil cooking spray
> 1½ tablespoons fresh lemon juice
> Dash of NoSalt
> ¼ teaspoon freshly ground black pepper (optional)

Combine ingredients, stirring with whisk. Cover and chill.

SALAD

> 3 cups romaine (or any) lettuce, chopped
> ¼ cucumber, thinly sliced
> ¼ cup red onion, sliced
> ¼ cup radishes, thinly sliced
> ½ tomato, sliced
> ¼ yellow pepper, chopped
> ¼ red pepper, chopped
> ¼ cup purple cabbage
> ¼ cup carrots, peeled and sliced
> ¼ cup broccoli florets
> 1 tablespoon Fiber One cereal (optional)

Place chopped lettuce in a large bowl; add rest of vegetables and toss to combine. Sprinkle with Fiber One cereal for texture if desired. Pour dressing over salad, tossing gently to coat or dress with your favorite store-bought salad dressing (go fat-free). My favorite is Ken's Raspberry Walnut Vinaigrette. Store-bought brands are not necessarily perfectly clean dressings, but they work in a pinch and are a far better option than any fast food you might end up eating.

CRUNCHY CABBAGE SLAW

Minutes to Prepare: 15   •   Number of Servings: 10   •   Yield: 2/3 cup

This is my family's all-time favorite way to eat their veggies, particularly when we barbecue at the lake. I've never had a complaint about this calcium- and vitamin-filled recipe—even from finicky kids. The dressing isn't perfect, but it's a much better choice than eating out. The warm dressing won't wilt the hardy cabbage, but it will make the leaves crisp-tender as they marinate. If you're in a hurry, buy the prepackaged slaw mix in your local market. When salad is done, you can warm the entire dish for a tasty treat. This slaw is fast, easy, and irresistibly delicious. A great side for your chicken breast.

3 cups green cabbage, shredded
1 cup red cabbage, shredded
1 cup red bell pepper, julienne cut
⅓ cup sunflower seeds or ⅓ cup Fiber One cereal (optional)
Ken's or Wishbone low-fat or fat-free Raspberry Walnut Vinaigrette
(warm it up for a special treat)

Pour dressing over cabbage and bell pepper in a large bowl; toss well. Sprinkle with NoSalt substitute if desired. Cover and chill two hours; stirring occasionally. Garnish with Fiber One cereal or sunflower seeds just before serving.

Green Apple Waldorf Salad

Minutes to Prepare: 15 • Number of Servings: 4

Eating an apple with or before dinner is one of the oldest tricks in the book when it comes to fighting hunger. Try this with a green apple, and you'll be amazed. This is a great salad for those days when you just can't get full. Mayo-free, it is a perfect blend of different flavors and textures to satisfy your sweet tooth.

> 1 large crisp apple such as Granny Smith or Gala
> 1 head Boston lettuce, trimmed, washed, and dried (may substitute fresh spinach)
> ½ cup shredded carrots
> ⅛ cup walnut halves (raw or toasted)
> 6 oz. cooked chicken breast (leftovers are great)
> ½ lemon, juiced
> ½ lemon zest, finely grated
> 2 tablespoons minced flat-leafed parsley for garnish(optional)

If you like toasted walnuts, preheat the oven to 350 degrees. Spread the nuts on a baking sheet and toast in the oven for 8 to 10 minutes. Cool and break up the nuts into small pieces.

Halve, core and cut the apples into ¾-inch pieces, leaving skin intact. Add apples and carrots to bowl and sprinkle with the lemon juice, then toss with fat-free raspberry walnut vinaigrette (or try pomegranate vinaigrette). Cover and refrigerate if not serving immediately.

When ready to serve, toss walnuts into the salad. Arrange the lettuce leaves (or spinach) on a large platter or divide them among four salad plates. Place the chicken and salad on the lettuce or spinach and serve.

CHINESE CHICKEN SALAD

Minutes to Prepare: 15 • Number of Servings: 4

It's undeniably one of the most popular salads in America, but did you know it's also one of the unhealthiest? Most versions of this that you'll find in national restaurant chains are nutritional disasters, bogged down by too much dressing and too many fried noodles. This lighter, cleaner version is true to Wolfgang Puck's original inspiration, but with about a third of the calories.

1 head Napa cabbage
½ head red cabbage
2 cups chopped or shredded cooked chicken (freshly grilled or store-bought rotisserie chicken)
½ tablespoon sugar
⅓ cup store-bought Asian vinaigrette
1 cup fresh cilantro leaves
¼ cup sliced almonds, toasted
1 cup canned mandarin oranges, drained
NoSalt and black pepper to taste

Slice cabbages in half lengthwise and remove cores. Then slice cabbage into thin strips. Toss with the sugar in a large bowl. If the chicken is cold, toss with a few tablespoons of vinaigrette and heat in a microwave at 50 percent power. Add chicken, cilantro, mandarins, almonds, and remaining vinaigrette to cabbage. Toss to combine. Season with NoSalt and pepper if desired.

MIRACLE IN A SALAD

Minutes to Prepare: 15 • Number of Servings: 4 to 6

This is one of the best and most eclectic salads you'll ever eat. When you're in the mood for change but don't feel like breaking your diet, it's good to try something different like this salad, with its combination of satisfying spicy and sweet flavors and hunger-curbing appeal. One of the first tricks I learned as a personal trainer was that if you can't get your clients to eat healthier, tell them to eat raspberries because they are full of fiber. Fiber acts like a sponge, helping transport fat and cholesterol out of the body. Choose the freshest baby greens you can find; they're higher in nutrients and offer an incredible taste.

1 cup fresh raspberries
¼ teaspoon NoSalt
4 cups loosely packed mixed leafy baby greens such as arugula or baby spinach
¼ teaspoon black pepper
¼ teaspoon crushed red pepper
½ cup snap peas
1 tablespoon sesame seeds
½ large red onion, thinly sliced
Olive oil spray
½ teaspoon honey
1 tablespoon finely chopped fresh sage (optional)

Simply spray the lettuce leaves with olive oil and gently toss the remaining ingredients. Can be served hot or cold. Make it a meal by adding shrimp, white fish, salmon, or chicken breast.

SLIMMING SAUCES AND THERMOGENIC DRESSINGS

Anyone can cook using butter and fats, but it's an art to cook lean and clean. All it takes is a little creativity and a few old Italian tricks. Your taste buds will adapt to not using butter and using less oil after a while. And you won't even notice that these delicious sauces are low- or no-fat. Most of the time, it's the sauce you crave, not what's underneath it. You'll be surprised how much your whole family will love these finger-licking good sauces.

These dressings are just as delicious as the fattier versions and great for making any kind of salad. Think out of the box when it comes to mixing tuna or salmon, shrimp, seafood, crab, chicken, or all vegetable salads if you're in a pinch. Don't underestimate those bagged lettuces when you're tight on time and your store's salad bar offers pick-up ready veggies for you to dunk. How easy is that for a weekday snack that boosts your metabolism and causes weight loss?

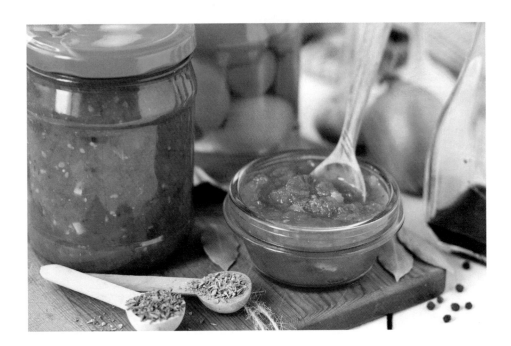

MELT-FAT MARINARA

Minutes to Prepare: 5 • Minutes to Cook: 10
Number of Servings: 4, if you're lucky

1 16-oz. can of crushed, no-salt-added tomatoes with basil, oregano, garlic, and onions al ready mixed in for convenience
1 teaspoon olive oil
1 tablespoon minced garlic or 1clove, minced
2 tablespoons fat-free chicken broth, if needed for a thinner sauce; use less for thicker
Olive oil spray, if needed

Lightly sauté garlic in olive oil. Remove pan from heat. Add crushed tomatoes and return to medium heat, then simmer. When cooking with less oil, watch food carefully as it may burn quickly. You can always add water or fat-free chicken broth to rehydrate if needed. There's no need to add more oil.

NO-COOK FAST AND EASY TOMATO SAUCE

Minutes to Prepare: 2 • Number of Servings: 2 to 3

Want faster sauce? Try my no-cook tomato sauce. This sauce is awesome, especially when you have fresh tomatoes from the garden or need a quick, delicious sauce to top off your clean foods. Get creative and try using all different kinds of tomatoes or whatever you have on hand.

    1 pint cherry or grape tomatoes
    Spray olive oil
    Garlic as desired (minced or fresh—your call)
    NoSalt and pepper to taste
    Fresh or dried basil (if desired)

Roughly chop the tomatoes and place in bowl. Stir in basil, spray with olive oil, NoSalt, and pepper. Allow to marinate 10 minutes if you can stand to wait to dig in. Otherwise, you're ready to go.

No time to make either sauce? Use your favorite salsa on top of your lean protein or over vegetables for a fast, delicious alternative. Still, nothing beats God's fresh ingredients, and you'll be a superstar at home with these.

TOP SECRET TUNA SAUCE
(THE VEGETARIAN MEAT SAUCE)

Minutes to Prepare: 5 • Minutes to Cook: 15 to 20 • Number of Servings: 2

I know, I know … tuna in a sauce? Trust me on this one; you are going to want to try this secret slimming sauce because it is delicious. This was my Aunt Rosemary's mom's recipe, and I couldn't believe it was tuna when I tried it for the first time. Adding tuna to your sauce not only makes it tastier, but it also makes it healthier. Tuna doesn't only thicken, it is one of the world's healthiest foods as it contains a rare form of selenium which plays a role as an important antioxidant binding together with mercury compounds and thus lowering the risk of mercury problems. The fact that tuna contains all of the essential amino acids, as well as omega-3s, gives you a good reason to eat it, not to mention that eating seafood helps you lose weight faster.

> 1 6½-oz. can tuna packed in water, drained
> ½ medium onion, chopped
> 1 6-oz. can of plum, no-salt-added tomatoes
> 1 tablespoon olive oil
> 1 tablespoon fat-free chicken broth
> 1 garlic clove crushed or 1 tablespoon minced garlic
> Pepper
> 3 anchovy fillets, rinsed (optional)

Heat oil in frying pan, add onions and sauté five minutes (add some broth if needed). Add garlic and cook until onions start to brown. Add anchovies if desired (crush them with spoon). Add tomatoes and simmer, covered, to form a sauce, about fifteen minutes.

Drain the tuna and break into large flakes. Add tuna to sauce with a little pepper (anchovies and tuna are already salty). Simmer, uncovered, for five minutes. Juices will evaporate and sauce will thicken.

This recipe can be made with boiled shrimp or clams, so get creative and leave the fattening meats out of it.

HERB SAUCE

Minutes to Prepare: 5 to 10 • Minutes to Cook: 5 • Number of Servings: 2 to 4

I come from an Italian family that can cook, but they never learned how to cook lean. I adore food—especially Italian food—so I took the time to travel in the Mediterranean to learn their way of cooking, which is the healthiest way to live lean for life. It was during my travels to Sicily that I learned how to make this herb sauce. It's more delicious than it sounds and goes great on top of fish and chicken or as a dipping sauce for vegetables. Try it, and I'm sure you'll love it, too. What makes this recipe unique is that it uses minimal oil, no butter, and is meat-, gluten-, and soy-free. It's free of just about everything except good taste.

2 ounces anchovies mashed
1 tablespoon capers
½ to 1 cup of chopped mushrooms
2 tablespoons parsley, chopped
2 garlic cloves, chopped
4 to 5 large basil leaves, chopped
½ teaspoon hot pepper flakes
⅓ cup of fat-free chicken broth
Olive oil spray

Mix all ingredients together, cook over low heat to warm up slowly. Stir and keep hot. Pour over fish, chicken, or your favorite vegetables.

This recipe is originally prepared with ¼ cup of black olives, ¼ cup of green olives, and ⅓ cup of olive oil. My family doesn't like olives, and I don't need the excess fat. Feel free to prepare it the way your family likes it best, and be prepared for a wild ride of flavor as this recipe will dazzle your taste buds.

PESTO
(PREPARE-TO-BOOST-YOUR-METABOLISM PESTO)

Minutes to Prepare: 5 • Number of Servings: 2 to 4

Everyone loves a good pesto sauce, but it's more fattening than a cheeseburger and French fries. There are many different ways to make it, but only this recipe is clean enough to help you get lean. Take the time to play with this recipe and make it yours—that's the secret to living lean. This sauce can be stored in a jar in the refrigerator for several weeks by adding more broth or a little olive oil to coat the top of the pesto. It's perfect for when you need a change from red sauce, and it doesn't have to be cooked if you're in a rush.

    1 cup fresh basil leaves, packed
    4 garlic cloves
    ¼ cup of grated Italian cheese (look for low-fat)
    1 cup of parsley, packed
    1 cup fat-free chicken broth
    ⅛ cup pignoli nuts (optional; omit if trying to lose weight)

Place basil, garlic, parsley, cheese and half the broth in a blender and blend together using low speed. Stop every few seconds to scrape the sides of the blender until everything is evenly mixed. Blend remaining broth in a steady stream. Continue blending until smooth in consistency.

Pour over fish or chicken or use as a vegetable dip.

BELL PEPPER COULIS SAUCE

Minutes to Prepare: 10 • Minutes to Cook: 20 • Makes 1 Pint

What's coulis? Pronounced "koo-lee," it is a simple sauce made of pureed vegetables, and it can be served hot or cold. This recipe for bell pepper coulis is great for company or on a hot night. Coulis makes a great veggie dip that's almost calorie-free so you can dip shrimp and vegetables all night. It can be made with red, yellow, or even orange peppers (not green) and makes a great soup, hot or cold.

2 to 3 large red, yellow, or orange bell peppers
2 ounces fat-free chicken broth or extra virgin olive oil
¼ cup vegetable stock or vegetable bouillon
Balsamic vinegar
NoSalt and pepper to taste (white pepper is awesome in this recipe)
2 tablespoons chopped shallots (optional)

Remove core, seeds, and membranes from the peppers and roughly chop them. Heat broth in a sauté pan over medium heat for one to two minutes. Add shallots if using and sauté until they are slightly translucent. Reduce heat to low and add the chopped pepper. Cover and sweat the vegetables for about 15 minutes or until tender.

Add a couple of tablespoons of stock and cook for another one to two minutes. Remove from heat and puree in blender. Caution: Be careful when blending hot liquids in blender as steam may pop lid off blender. Start on slow speed with lid slightly ajar, slowly increasing blender speed.

Add vinegar. Adjust consistency with remaining stock and season to taste with NoSalt and pepper.

Mustard Sauce and Dressing
(Aka Metabolic-Boosting Mustard Sauce)

Minutes to Prepare: 5 • Minutes to Cook: 5 • Serves: 4 to 6

While mustard sauce is usually a cream sauce, this one is lean, clean, and oh-so-delicious. It's awesome with eggs or over vegetables, fish, or chicken, and makes an awesome salad dressing. I learned about this sauce/dressing from my bodybuilder friends who live to be lean and will not eat fatty foods. Tangy mustard sauce has practically no fat or carbs and is low-sodium to boot.

Olive oil spray
2 tablespoons prepared mustard of choice (Dijon is best)
2 minced garlic cloves or 2 teaspoons jarred
¼ cup balsamic or red wine vinegar
¾ teaspoon chopped rosemary (optional)
¼ cup fat-free, low-sodium chicken broth
NoSalt and pepper to taste

Spray pan with olive oil over medium heat. Add minced garlic and sauté 30 seconds, stirring constantly. Stir in vinegar, broth, and Dijon mustard. Bring to boil. Cook until reduced to one quarter cup (about five minutes), stirring occasionally. Stir in rosemary and black pepper.

For a really special day, add two tablespoons of maple syrup for extra yumminess.

TOP FIVE Ways to Eat Your Veggies:
1) Chopped in raw salads or shredded to make veggie slaw
2) Dunked raw in your favorite clean dressing
3) Cut a head of lettuce in half, grill it, then top with dressing.
4) Add water and your favorite seasoning to make vegetable soup.
5) Pureed and added to your favorite sauce or dressing to thicken it—not your waist

---

TANGY MUSTARD DRESSING

Need a delicious salad dressing when you're out with friends? This salad dressing is the easiest and most delicious. Best of all, it can be made anywhere, anytime—even at a diner. Simply mix together mustard and vinegar (any kind you can get your hands on) and add one packet of Equal, if needed. NoSalt and pepper to taste. Voila! You have a delicious fat-free dressing. No more excuses.

SEXY SALSA DRESSING

Minutes to Prepare: 15 • Minutes to Cook: 20 • Serves: 6

This simple dressing is not simple when it comes to taste and the big bang it packs in flavor. Use it on salads, over fish, or as a stir-fry mix-in. Always remember you can dip boring veggies or dull, dry lean protein in these dressings, making them more appealing. Everyone loves fondue style. Sexy salsa is great as a salad dressing and makes a great sauce for shrimp salad and/or dip. I think every refrigerator should have a stash of this—it's delicious and kids love to help make it too.

4 large ripe tomatoes, cut into bite-size pieces
1 bunch cilantro, stems cut off and leaves coarsely chopped
1 large green bell pepper, cut into bite-size pieces
1 large red bell pepper, cut into bite-size pieces
3 green onions, chopped
½ sweet red onion, chopped
1 lime, juiced
½ teaspoon NoSalt to taste

In a large salad bowl, lightly mix the tomatoes, cilantro, green and red bell peppers, green onions, and sweet red onion until thoroughly combined. Squeeze lime juice over salad. Sprinkle with NoSalt to serve. Can't make it fast enough? Use canned, chopped tomatoes. And if you like it hotter, add finely chopped jalapeños.

THAI DIPPING SAUCE OR SALAD DRESSING

Minutes to Prepare: 5 • Minutes to Cook: 5 • Serves: 2

This sauce will get your kids and whole family to devour whatever healthy food you're trying to disguise. I'll let you in on a little secret: I hated vegetables until I realized that eating them helped me lose weight, and I hated the fact that my plate was bare unless I filled it with veggies. The secret to my vegetable eating success is finding delicious, creative ways to enjoy them. This is one of my favorites, and it goes great on chicken or as a salad dressing—it's especially good for dipping.

2 tablespoons PB2 peanut butter powder*
1 tablespoon low-sodium soy sauce
1 tablespoon water
⅛ teaspoon garlic powder
¼ teaspoon pepper (ground is best)
1 teaspoon Splenda brown sugar
⅛ teaspoon sesame oil
⅛ teaspoon Szechuan chili sauce (optional)

Blend all ingredients well and serve. Refrigerate any remaining sauce. How easy is that?

*PB2 by Bell Plantation (bellplantation.com) is a peanut butter powder available in many stores and online.

BE LEAN BLUE CHEESE

Minutes to Prepare: 5 • Serves: 4 to 6 salads

We all need help when it comes to enjoying clean food, and blue cheese is a helper that just about everyone loves, especially for veggie dipping, on top of dry turkey burgers, or simply drizzled on grilled romaine lettuce (my favorite) for a fast, easy, weight-loss friendly, and scrumptious salad. However, blue cheese also dumps about 30 grams of fat on your salad (because it contains oil, mayonnaise, cheese, and buttermilk), which puts you well over the 15 to 20 grams of fat you need to stay under when trying to lose weight. Try this lighter version instead!

¼ cup blue cheese, finely chopped
½ cup Greek yogurt (choose one with the fewest calories and zero fat) for a thicker dressing, or use buttermilk for a lighter version that's thinner
Juice of ½ lemon (try it with a Meyer lemon)
1 tablespoon white vinegar
¼ teaspoon NoSalt
Black pepper to taste
Sprinkle of garlic powder
Sprinkle of onion powder
Dash of Equal or Splenda

Finely chop and break apart blue cheese into tiny crumbles. Combine blue cheese, Greek yogurt, lemon juice, and vinegar in a bowl (better yet, make it in a jar so you can save the remaining dressing for later) and mix well.

Add all of the other seasonings and stir well with a fork until cheese is no longer clumping. The secret to disguising this healthy version is to make sure it's mixed well.

You can adjust to desired thickness by using thicker yogurts for a thicker dressing, or adding water (one tablespoon at a time) if you prefer it thinner until you reach the thickness you prefer. On special occasions, try a drizzle of honey in it. Want more pizzazz? Add a dash of hot sauce; it's practically calorie-free.

FAT-BLASTING CAESAR DRESSING

Minutes to Prepare: 5 • Serves: 4 to 6 salads

Who doesn't adore Caesar dressing? I could live on Caesar salads every day, and I did at first. This was one of my big mistakes when I started eating healthy and found I still wasn't losing weight. You know why? Depending on what you put in your salad, it can have more calories than a cheeseburger and fries combined. I spent my life researching ways to make recipes leaner, but leaner without tasting yummy wasn't good enough. I picked the brains of the chefs at Martha Stewart's and asked all of my chef friends (while waiting on TV sets, I am in the back room picking brains of awesome people like Chef Big Daddy Aaron McCargo, Jr.) to find out their secrets and came up with this fast and easy lean Caesar dressing. If you're pressed for time, you could use the lowest-calorie bottled Caesar dressing you can find in your store, but there is nothing like making this from scratch.

⅓ cup grated reduced-fat Parmesan cheese (I prefer Parmigiano Reggiano)
¼ cup fresh lemon juice (Meyer lemons make it better)
1 small garlic clove
½ teaspoon Dijon mustard
2 anchovy fillets*
1 tablespoon fat-free chicken broth (or 1 tablespoon extra virgin olive oil if you can afford the calories)
5 tablespoons fat-free plain Greek yogurt (lowest calorie you can find)

In a food processor add the cheese, lemon juice, garlic clove, Dijon mustard, and the anchovies. Blend in food processor for 15 to 20 seconds. Add the oil and yogurt and blend for additional 15 seconds, and there you have it. Hold the croutons.

*Not an anchovy fan? Leave them out, but they are what make this dressing so awesome.

GREEN AND LEAN CUCUMBER RANCH DRESSING

Minutes to Prepare: 10 • Serves: 6 salads

Ranch is one of the most popular dressings in the United States, a staple at every salad bar. But it is horrible for you, unless you eat this green and lean version. Kids love it and moms approve—and so will your skinny jeans. Unlike other ranch dressings that contain everything that's bad for you, this version is light and very refreshing, thanks to the thermogenic cucumbers that help blast the metabolism and keep calories low.

½ cup low-fat buttermilk
¼ cup fat-free plain Greek yogurt (look for the lowest calorie and fat at your supermarket)
1 small cucumber, peeled and seeded (or you can leave seeds in for texture—I do)
1 clove garlic
3 tablespoons fresh or dried parsley
¼ cup scallions (optional)
Juice of half a lemon
⅛ teaspoon garlic powder
NoSalt and pepper to taste

Combine all ingredients in a blender or food processor and blend for 15 to 30 seconds until desired consistency is reached. For extra oomph, add a dash of horseradish.

HALLELUJAH HONEY MUSTARD, THE SIMPLEST SKINNY DRESSING EVER

Minutes to Prepare: 10 • Serves: 1 to 2 salads

Honey mustard has always been one of my favorites, naturally, because it's sweet. This dressing is delicious and good for you—not to mention it's fast and easy and kills the bottled stuff you can buy. Kids love it and will eat their veggies and chicken if you make this dunk sauce. I love it after a day in the country with the kids when we pick up a local bottle of honey and fresh vegetables at a farm stand. It's amazing how the small things like this can motivate kids to eat healthy. Get them involved and make a day of learning about honey and what makes it different when it's from your local area. They will be fascinated and want to eat it. Did you know pure honey is antibacterial and antifungal, helps reduce coughs and throat irritations, and may ease gastrointestinal disorders? Don't forget though that honey is a sugar, and all sugar can elevate blood sugar levels no matter how healthy it is. It is a good idea to include honey with a protein to help blunt blood sugar levels from rising. Try to eat this on the weekends to keep things balanced.

  1 tablespoon Dijon mustard
  1 teaspoon honey

Mix together and eat. It's that simple.

Want it sugar free? Omit honey, add a dash of water to thin out and add one packet of Splenda for a sugar-free version.

If you need a bigger batch for company, add buttermilk (skim milk works, too). Adjust the mustard and honey to taste as desired. If you want a thicker version, process some radishes in a food processor, and they will thicken it right up without anyone even knowing you added them. Radishes, by the way, are virtually calorie-free.

MOJITO LIME DRESSING

Minutes to Prepare: 5 • Serves: 4

This is delicious on a hot summer night on just about anything from salads to a dip for veggies to topping for your Lean Tuna Burgers. It has a little nonfat mayo in it, and when I make it I use it sparingly, if at all, saving the full mayonnaise amount for special occasions. Try this when you need a change over your salad or mix cabbage or broccoli (try pre-shredded store-bought bags when you're in a hurry) with it for a delicious lime slaw.

½ cup fat-free mayonnaise
2 tablespoons chopped mint
1 tablespoon fresh lime juice (bottled is fine, too)

Combine ingredients and stir until blended.

MELT-FAT MEDITERRANEAN

Minutes to Prepare: 5 • Serves: 1

This dressing is a classic all across the Mediterranean, but it only becomes lean when you reduce olive oil amounts or, better yet, use spray olive oil instead so you can control portions. Melt-Fat Mediterranean dressing is simply delicious and a great way to show off the taste of fresh vegetables and seafood—the cleaner the food, the better. It goes with everything. Just be careful with the olive oil, and you'll be fine.

1 teaspoon high-quality extra virgin olive oil (look for cold-pressed) or olive oil spray for better portion control

Juice from one lemon (Meyer lemons make it extra special)

Sprinkle of lemon zest

Dash of NoSalt and pepper

Simply mix everything together and use this to dress your salads as well as for other cooking needs. It is the simplest dressing ever and the best tasting.

Don't Have Time for Homemade Dressing?

When all else fails, go for your favorite bottled dressing from your local supermarket. My favorite is Paul Newman's. To make it leaner, I dilute it with vinegar to reduce the fat and salt. Always look for a bottle with the lowest calories, carbohydrates, and salt you can find. And don't ever forget to be on the lookout for sugar. Yes, dressings can be full of it.

The Best To-Go and On-the-Go Meals

Whether you're an office worker, student, or a harried mom running around to doctor appointments and school meetings, most lunchtimes (or meals on the go) consist of being held hostage to a handful of fast-food and sit-down chains. This is exactly why a quality whey protein shake makes losing weight so easy. All you have to do is drink your nutrition and go on with your day.

Brown-bagging is inevitable at times. Whether you're with family at the beach, in your backyard by the pool, or at a ballgame, you need to be ready with the right foods. Lunch or any meal on the go still needs to consist of a small serving of lean protein and vegetables if you're serious about boosting your metabolism. Try these fast, easy, grab-and-go lunches (when you can't drink a shake), and you'll never be caught downing a drive-thru milkshake for lunch again.

1. Make lettuce wraps instead of using bread. Simply wrap your favorite protein in a lettuce leaf. It's what celebs do.
2. Make it a salad (vegetable salads too)—of course, without all the croutons, cheese, bacon, yolks, beans, or full-fat dressings.
3. Slim down and fill up with soup. Soup can be enjoyed hot or cold depending on the season.

It's easy to make lean, light salads. Simply combine tuna, egg whites, chicken, or salmon; even sliced turkey from the deli works in a pinch. All of these ingredients can be mixed with the dressings in this book.

If you're really in a rush, try these simpler varieties:
Start with a lettuce wrap, a base of lettuce leaves chopped up, or you can use your favorite vegetables if you prefer—as long as you don't use bread. Simply mix the items below with one of the thermogenic dressings or use a simple, store-bought fat-free mustard, salsa, or the cleanest bottled dressing you can find. Remember to look for fat-free or the lowest fat available, low or no carbs, little or no sugar (yes, dressings have sugar in them), and, of course, low sodium.

1. Lean Protein: Tuna, salmon, chicken breast, crab meat, egg whites, or two to three slices of low-sodium deli turkey
2. Other Mix-ins:
   - Add your favorite fat-free salsa, Dijon mustard, or any fat-free mustard.
   - Add one half to one cup of your favorite frozen mixed veggies and season with Mrs. Dash, McCargo's Signature Blend, or your favorite seasoning.

- Add fresh lemon juice, Dijon mustard, and garlic paste (made by finely chopping a fresh clove and smashing it into a paste), and season with fresh pepper.
- Mix veggie/tuna mixture together until well incorporated. Taste. Add NoSalt if necessary.
- Add crunchy veggies like carrots, celery, onion, or think out of the box and add pineapple or apple chunks to your chicken salads.

More Slimming Salad Alternatives:

* BLUE CHEESE BLUES: Slice a head of iceberg lettuce in half and drizzle with Be Lean Blue Cheese over the big chunk.

* THAI: Buy a container of your favorite greens and three ounces of chicken breast (canned is fine); drizzle with Thai salad dressing and top with a few slivered almonds. Great with chopped scallions.

* CAESAR: Toss three cups of romaine with shrimp, salmon, or chicken breast.

* SEXY SALSA SALAD: This is a great chopped salad. Chop three cups of your favorite lettuce and three ounces of shrimp or chicken chunks and toss with Sexy Salsa dressing.

* FAJITA SALAD: Make lean fajitas (sauté three ounces cooked chicken breast with assorted peppers, NoSalt, pepper, and olive oil spray) and top your salad. No dressing needed. Let the juices drip onto the salad.

SNEAK IN A LITTLE WHEY PROTEIN POWDER TO BOOST METABOLISM

The following are recipes I use to add variety and fun while sneaking extra protein into my diet ... it's easy, and your kids will love it, too!

WHEY PROTEIN PANCAKES

2 scoops of your favorite flavor of whey protein powder
⅛ cup of water

Place protein powder in a bowl and add just enough water that the mixture has a consistency similar to pancake batter (it should be slightly lumpy). Pour the mixture into a nonstick skillet sprayed with nonstick cooking spray, and cook on medium heat, one to two minutes per side. Top with cinnamon or the zero-calorie syrup of your choice (I like Walden's). Try experimenting with vanilla, almond, or coconut extracts to get lots of flavor without the calories.

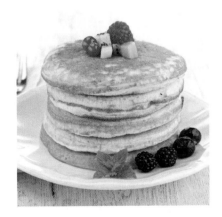

TURBOCHARGING, PROTEIN-PACKED JELL-O

> 2 scoops of your favorite protein powder
> 1 package sugar free Jell-O (any flavor)

Make Jell-O according to directions. Before setting to gel, add the protein powder. Let stand to set. I always have this on hand so I can CHOW whenever I need to.

WARM METABOLIC DRINKS

In the mood for something warm and cozy? You can mix these in a blender or use a frother for a real treat.

SKINNY HOT CHOCOLATE: Add 1 to 2 scoops of chocolate whey protein powder to warm (not hot) water.

LEAN LATTE: Add 1 to 2 scoops of vanilla whey protein powder to 6 ounces warm coffee and sprinkle with cinnamon.

METABOLIC MOCHACHINO: Add 1 to 2 scoops of your favorite whey protein powder to 6 ounces of warm coffee.

HOT PEPPERMINT MOCHA: Add 1 to 2 scoops of chocolate whey protein powder and 3 drops of mint extract to 6 ounces of warm coffee.

WARM ALMOND AB BLAST: Add 1 to 2 scoops of vanilla or chocolate whey protein powder and 3 drops of almond extract to 6 ounces of warm coffee.

I WANNA BE LEAN ICE CREAM

There are thousands of options to choose from when it comes to making lean ice cream. Choose the flavor you're craving and enjoy. (P.S. They make great shakes, too!)

PEANUT BUTTER AND CHOCOLATE DREAM

> 1 to 2 scoops of chocolate whey protein powder
> 1 teaspoon peanut butter
> ½ cup water
> 4 ice cubes

Fill food processor with water and ice cubes and blend until the ice is crushed into a fine snow. Scrape down sides of processor. Add whey protein powder and peanut butter. Mix for two to three minutes. Then serve and enjoy.

STRAWBERRY TRUFFLE ICE CREAM

>2 scoops strawberry whey protein powder
>3 teaspoons sugar-free white chocolate pudding mix
>½ cup water
>4 ice cubes

Fill food processor with water and ice cubes and blend until the ice is crushed into a fine snow. Scrape down sides of processor. Add whey protein powder and white chocolate pudding mix. Process for two to three minutes, then serve and enjoy.

VERY VANILLA ICE CREAM

>2 scoops vanilla whey protein powder
>1½ envelopes of unflavored gelatin
>¼ cup cold water
>1 teaspoon vanilla extract
>¾ cup boiling water

Sprinkle gelatin over cold water to soften. Add vanilla and boiling water. Stir to dissolve gelatin. Refrigerate until mixture starts to set. Mix at high speed until mixture becomes frothy. Add whey protein powder and beat at high speed for 10 minutes. Pour into two one-pint plastic containers and freeze.

COOKIES FOR WEIGHT LOSS

Who doesn't love a good cookie? Follow this recipe and enjoy guilt-free cookie enjoyment.

>2 scoops of your favorite whey protein powder
>1 egg white

Mix egg white and whey protein powder in bowl. Add water to the mixture until it forms a doughy substance. Spray a bowl with nonstick cooking spray and add batter. Place in a microwave and heat 15 to 45 seconds, depending on the power of your microwave.

TRY THESE FLAVOR BOOSTERS

Adding flavor doesn't mean you need to add calories. Try experimenting with the following flavor boosters for a calorie-free flavor punch.

EXTRACTS: Vanilla, Almond, Coconut, Banana, Mint
PEANUT BUTTER: Add a teaspoon to satisfy your craving.
Sugar-Free, Fat-Free Jell-O: Try every flavor under the sun until you fall in love with one. My favorite flavor is lemon.

DECADENT DESSERTS

Are you like me? Do you live for dessert? I am more than willing to give up the carbs; I think they are sadly overrated. But I cannot imagine living without dessert. The good news: You don't have to. *The Metabolism Solution* is specifically designed to boost your metabolism so you burn more calories, even at rest, which leaves some room in your caloric budget for Real Life Indulgences—for those moments when you just have to have something delicious. Dessert is why we drink the shake in the morning—it allows us a little room for real life.

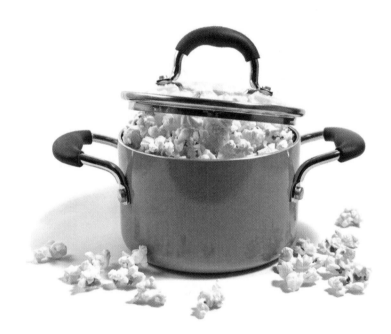

KETTLE CORN

Minutes to Prepare: 5 • Minutes to Cook: 5 • Number of Servings: 2
Serving Size: 3 Cups

Popcorn is a whole grain and full of fiber. Add some whey protein powder to it, and you have a terrific metabolic-boosting, faster-fat-burning snack. Its sweet and salty flavors work for just about everyone.

6 cups air-popped popcorn or whatever popped corn you have
⅛ teaspoon NoSalt or salt substitute (Can't find one? Use salt.)
2 packets of Stevia or Splenda Butter-flavored cooking spray

Combine ingredients in a bowl. With the back of a teaspoon, crush mixture until it is like powder. Doing this makes it easier to sprinkle and the salt isn't as concentrated. Try whirring the seasonings in a food processor to crush into smaller particles and then store them in a shaker for faster, easier use.

When your corn is finished popping, give it a spray with butter-flavored cooking spray and quickly sprinkle your homemade kettle corn seasoning. Toss the corn until seasoning is evenly distributed.

CINNAMON SUGAR: Add ¼ teaspoon cinnamon
CHOCOLATE POPCORN: Add 1 teaspoon to 1 tablespoon chocolate whey protein powder
PIZZA POPCORN: Add desired amount of grated reduced-fat Parmesan cheese, 1 teaspoon dried oregano, 1 tablespoon finely chopped sun-dried tomatoes, ¼ teaspoon red pepper flakes, ¼ teaspoon garlic powder

PROTEIN PEANUT BUTTER BLISS BALLS

Minutes to Prepare: 5 • Minutes to Cook: 10 • Serving Size: 1 ball

This has got to be one of the best weekend cheat foods on the planet. Thank God I don't have time to make this often, but when I do, I am sure to make extra and freeze them for those need-one-now moments. (Don't we all have them?) They are easy to prepare and healthy enough to eat when you need a fix. This should make enough servings to last a couple of weeks. Store the remainder in a Tupperware container in the fridge. Remember, this is a weekend cheat food, unless you can only eat one. These peanut butter balls are rich in calories, but the whey gives you high-quality protein, the oats give you fiber and low-glycemic carbs, the honey boosts your immune system, and the peanut butter provides healthy unsaturated fats and antioxidants. Want to go really clean? Skip the oats.

> 2 scoops chocolate or vanilla whey protein powder
> ¼ cup honey
> 1 cup natural peanut butter
> ¾ cup raw oats

Mix all the ingredients in a large bowl. Powder your hands with some flour (to prevent stickiness) and form into one-inch balls and place on a baking sheet. Bake at 375 degrees for five to ten minutes.

For a special occasion treat: Dip them in melted dark chocolate and roll them in shredded coconut, sprinkles, or nuts. They make great gifts.

RICH COCOA SORBETO

Minutes to Prepare: 10 • Minutes to Freeze: 20 • Servings: 4

One thing we all crave at one time or another is ice cream. Why? It's mood food. Ice cream is one of the biggest diet destroyers. To help you get your fix without sabotaging all the work you do on The Metabolism Solution plan, I created this sorbeto that, unlike ice cream, isn't loaded with fat or sugar so it's low in calories and carbs. My sorbeto has 1 gram of fat and 25 carbs. You can keep losing weight even if you eat it—dare I say it—every day? You can thank researchers in part for removing some of the guilt from this guilty pleasure. Studies have shown that chocolate, particularly dark chocolate with at least 70 percent cocoa, can help protect you from heart disease and some cancers while boosting your immune system thanks to plant chemicals called flavonoids. Ounce for ounce, cocoa powder has a higher concentration of age-fighting antioxidants than other foods. Most chocolate desserts are loaded with sugar, heavy cream, butter, and other heavy ingredients that neutralize cocoa's healthy effects. Not this one.

    1 cup natural cocoa powder
    1¾ cups of water
    ¾ cup honey (substitute with ¾ cup Splenda or Stevia for even cleaner version)
    ½ teaspoon NoSalt
    1½ teaspoons vanilla extract

Place cocoa into small saucepan. Slowly whisk in ¾ cup water until cocoa is dissolved and there are no lumps. Whisk in honey or sweetener, NoSalt, and remaining 1 cup of water. Stir over medium heat until mixture begins to boil. Remove from heat. Stir in vanilla.

When cool, pour mixture into the canister of an ice cream maker and freeze according to manufacturer's instructions; or you can freeze mixture in a bowl, process in a food processor, then refreeze until sorbet is set.

My trick? Add 1 cup of chocolate whey protein powder in place of the cocoa to help keep your metabolism revved—it makes it even yummier. Any of the shake recipes that you love can also be made into sorbet. Simply freeze them. Allow them to thaw just enough so you can easily eat them with a spoon.

Rocky Road High Protein Fudge Bars

Minutes to Prepare: 10 • Minutes to Freeze: 20 • Serving: 1 "bar"

This will be your new favorite, healthy "cheat day" dessert. This "fudge" is full of lean protein, fiber, and calcium; honey is great for B vitamins and boosting your immunity. You'll never eat regular fudge again. Make extra for when your sweet tooth calls.

1 cup chocolate whey protein powder
½ cup Nutella Spread
¼ to ½ cup marshmallows
¼ cup honey (substitute ¼ cup Stevia or Splenda if desired)
¼ cup rolled oats

Equipment Needed:

Freezer or ice pack
Heavy spatula
Blender
Bowl
10 pieces aluminum foil cut ½ the width of the roll x 6 inches

In a large mixing bowl, mix rolled oats (uncooked) and 1 cup chocolate whey protein powder until blended. Add Nutella and honey and mix until thoroughly blended and the mixture holds its shape. Add marshmallows until desired look and taste is met.

Form a patty one-inch thick or make a candy bar shape using the spatula; place on aluminum foil. Put in freezer and chill until frozen.

When nicely frozen, remove and cut into smaller bars of desired size. Keep chilled until just before eating if possible so the cold bars and patties keep their shape (freezing also keeps them from spoiling).

Variations:
  • Add one banana to the mixture to make the texture chewier.
  • Add dry spices such as cinnamon and nutmeg.
  • Add walnuts or almonds.
  • Add a shot of coconut or vanilla flavoring (add extra oats to compensate for added liquid).

APPLE WHEY GOOD CRISPILICIOUS

Minutes to Prepare: 10 • Minutes to Cook: 20 to 30 • Servings: 4

Great to have on hand when company is coming. The vanilla whey protein powder adds a metabolic-boosting protein punch. This dessert has fiber to help keep things regular and apples have been known to suppress appetite. Keep plenty of apples on hand so you are never without.

BASE

3 apples, cored and sliced
½ cup applesauce, unsweetened
1½ teaspoons lemon juice
1 teaspoon Splenda
1 scoop vanilla whey protein powder
1 teaspoon Splenda brown sugar
½ teaspoon cinnamon

TOPPING

1 cup oatmeal
2 tablespoons Splenda brown sugar
1 scoop vanilla whey protein powder
2 tablespoons Smart Balance (optional; you can use a sprinkle of water for moisture)

Mix together base ingredients and spoon into a greased (use spray) cooking dish. Combine the topping mix and crumble over the base.

Bake at 350 degrees for 20 to 30 minutes or until golden brown. You can also cook this in the microwave—cooking times vary, so keep an eye on it.

Serve with one scoop of vanilla nonfat, sugar-free yogurt or Very Vanilla Sorbeto for special occasions. Just as good with a cup of vanilla tea.

COCOA MERINGUES

Minutes to Prepare: 10 • Cooking Time: 2 hours • Servings: 10 (4 per serving)

I'm obsessed with meringues, and these little cookies fulfill the craving for something sweet without the guilt. They do have a little bit of sugar, but we all have those moments when we just need something yummy.

3 egg whites
⅛ teaspoon cream of tartar
⅓ cup sugar (superfine, if possible)
¼ teaspoon almond extract
2 tablespoons unsweetened cocoa

Preheat oven to 200 degrees. Cover a baking sheet with parchment paper.

Place egg whites and cream of tartar in large bowl; beat with mixer at high speed until foamy. Add sugar, one tablespoon at a time, beating until stiff peaks form. Beat in extract.

Spoon mixture into pastry bag or Zip Lock plastic bag with one corner snipped to a ¼ inch-sized opening. Pipe 40 1-inch rounds ¼ inch apart on prepared baking sheet. Bake at 200 degrees Farenheit for two hours.

Turn off oven, cool meringues in closed oven at least one hour. Carefully remove meringues from paper and toss them with cocoa in zip-top plastic bag to coat.

HOMEMADE BAKED CINNAMON APPLE CHIPS

Minutes to Prepare: 5 to 10 • Cooking Time: 2 to 3 hours • Servings: 4

Do you crave crunch? This one's for you. As you know, apples are one of my top snack suggestions and make the Top Ten list of snacks on every diet on the planet from Atkins to Paleo. I cleaned up the usual version and made this one sugar-free, which not only makes this recipe better for your metabolism, but it also makes it a great snack for kids, too. It contains only two ingredients, so it's very simple. Make sure to use apples that have a great flavor to begin with, ones that you would enjoy eating raw. Otherwise the chips might turn out bitter, and you'll be wondering why.

> 1 to 2 apples (I use Honeycrisp)
> 1 teaspoon cinnamon

Preheat oven to 200 degrees.

Using a sharp knife or mandoline, slice apples thinly. Discard seeds and core. Prepare a baking sheet with parchment paper and arrange apple slices on it without overlapping. Sprinkle cinnamon over apples.

Bake for approximately 1 hour, then flip. Continue baking for one to two hours, flipping occasionally, until the apple slices are no longer moist. Store in airtight container. The baking time varies, depending on your oven and how thick the apple slices were cut. You want to cut them as thinly as possible. Usually, mandolines work better for this sort of work, but I have found that the whole apple can be too wide for a mandoline. I use a sharp knife, which is why the thickness varies a teeny bit.

My Trick: I sprinkle the slices with a little metabolism-boosting vanilla whey protein powder to add sweetness instead of sugar.

HOMEMADE FROZEN STRAWBERRY POPS

Minutes to Prepare: 3 • Freezing Time: 2 hours • Servings: 4

Of course the best way to lose weight fast and enjoy a frozen treat is to freeze your protein shake. Frozen pops are great to have around a house with kids (and all their friends). I love these in the summer when it's boiling outside; it's a delicious way to get more fluids in.

  3 cups fat-free plain Greek yogurt
  2 cups frozen unsweetened strawberries
  2 teaspoons vanilla extract
  2 tablespoons of honey, agave nectar or Splenda

Combine yogurt, strawberries, vanilla extract, and sweetener of choice in blender. Process until smooth. Pour the mixture into four ice-pop molds or paper cups. Place ice cream stick in the middle of each cup and freeze for two hours or until solid. To serve, remove from molds or peel away paper cup.

Variation: For a truly decadent frozen pop, replace strawberries with banana and ½ scoop of chocolate whey protein powder. Unbelievably good!

ESPRESSO GRANITA

Minutes to Prepare: 10   •   Freezing Time: 2 hours or more   •   Servings: 4

Forget driving into town for a scoop of fattening ice cream that will set you back a half-day's worth of calories. Frozen granitas are just as satisfying as ice cream and very easy to make. Your metabolism and wallet will thank you, as you'll save lots of calories and money. Unlike most versions of granitas, this one is sugar-free and extremely low-calorie—it's practically free food.

> 2 cups espresso or very strong brewed coffee, warmed
> ½ cup of Splenda or Truvia
> ½ cup shaved dark chocolate
> Light whipped topping (optional)

Combine espresso or coffee with Splenda or Truvia and stir until dissolved. Pour mixture into shallow metal baking pan and place in freezer.

After 20 minutes, just as the mix begins to freeze, remove the pan from the freezer and use a fork to scrape the ice crystals developing on the surface into a serving cup and enjoy! Scraping will help you achieve a light, creamy granita rather than a chunky, icy one. Return the pan to freezer and repeat this step every 30 minutes until granita is entirely frozen.

To serve, I scoop it into a chilled wine glass. For special occasions, I layer each serving, alternating between granita and light whipped topping with chocolate shavings.

FIVE

YOUR WORKOUT MAY BE SLOWING YOUR METABOLISM

These days, there are hundreds of exercise programs for you to choose from. You can work out 24 hours a day at the never-closing gym; you can do cold yoga and hot yoga, train like a Navy S.E.A.L., stretch like a ballet dancer, twirl around a stripper's pole, and "whatever-cize" away the fat. Where do you start?

You know you can lose weight without exercise if you can control your food intake. So why bother at all? I'll tell you why: to feel good. You want to tone up your arms for the dress you're wearing to your son's graduation. You want to be able to run after your toddler without getting out of breath. You want to sleep better. You want to find an outlet for the stress in your life. You want to move without your body aching. You want to reduce your risk of heart disease, high blood pressure, cancer, and diabetes. Need I go on?

Oh, and did I mention that exercise can turbocharge your metabolism? It's a sad fact that as you age, your metabolic rate (how quickly your body burns calories for fuel) slows down. Starting at about age 25, the average, physically inactive person's metabolism declines between 5 and 10 percent per decade, which accumulates to a decline of between 20 to 40 percent over an adult life span. However, there is some good news for those who continue physical activity their whole lives: only a 0.3 percent metabolic decline per decade. Isn't that a good reason to keep moving? If your current fitness program isn't working, needs a jump-start, leaves you hurting, or is nonexistent, you've come to the right place.

THE SLOW METABOLISM TEST

Do you have a hard time losing weight? Do you feel flabby, fatigued, and fat? You may be struggling with a sluggish metabolism. The good news is that no matter how much damage has been done from constant yo-yo dieting, eating the wrong foods, or lack of exercise, it can be fixed. How do you know if your metabolism is slow? Chances are that if you're reading this, you already know the answer to that question; but I suggest that you take The Metabolism Test to give you the answers you need to solve your weight-loss problems once and for all. It can be fixed, and *The Metabolism Solution* will show you how.

The Metabolism Test—Please answer with a simple yes or no.

- Do you have a hard time losing weight?
- Do you struggle with cravings for carbohydrate foods and sugar?
- Do you have to starve yourself in order to lose an ounce?

- Do you exercise but still can't lose weight?
- Do you carry excess pounds and fat, specifically around your midsection, hips and thighs?
- Do you have cellulite covering your body and on areas where cellulite typically does not go?
- Are you tired and sluggish most of the time?
- Are you female?
- Are you over 30?
- Have you been chronically stressed for more than 30 days?
- Do you drink more than one drink per week?
- Were your parents or grandparents overweight?
- Have you gone through peri-menopause or menopause?
- Are you considered short? (Under five feet, four inches)?
- Is your waist size more than 35 inches (women) or 40 inches (men)?
- Do you have any of the following medical conditions that you are aware of?
  » High blood pressure (systolic over 130 or Diastolic over 85)?
  » High cholesterol?
  » Low HDL (good) cholesterol?
  » Allergies?
  » High blood sugar (110 or higher)?
  » High triglycerides (150 or higher)?
  » Depression/anxiety?
  » Seizures?
  » Do you sleep less than seven hours per night?
  » Have you been told that you are hypo- or hypothyroid by a doctor?
  » Do you take medications to treat any of these ailments?
  » Do you retain water or feel bloated often?
  » Do you have at least one bowel movement every day?
  » Do you have food sensitivities? Gluten? Dairy? Fish?
  » Have you gained more than 10 pounds in the last two years?
  » Have you lost weight and regained it more than once in the last two years?
  » Do you think your metabolism is slow?

If you answered YES to five or more of these questions, your metabolism is slow and needs to be boosted in order for you to lose weight and feel great. The more YES's, the more critical it is. Even if you answered YES to fewer than five questions, it's still a good idea to add the suggestions outlined in these pages to keep your metabolism moving. *The Metabolism Solution* is the answer to losing weight and preventing you from gaining weight as you age.

BOOSTING A SLOW METABOLISM WITH METABOLIC EXERCISE

Not all exercise is created equal. Metabolic Exercise is key to revving up your calorie-burning engine. Simply put, metabolic training uses eight to ten specific multitasking moves (some using dumbbells) to work all the major muscle groups in every thirty-minute workout no more than three times a week. You read it right: not every day, but three days a week. Each move includes at least two large muscle groups per move, and they always include a leg move so you triple your calorie burn in half the time. That's intensity. And there's no rest between moves either. This is combined with daily aerobic walking I call the Metabolic Core Walk. You don't have to do all the moves in one session. You can break up a metabolic workout and do a little at a time throughout the day in your own home or even at an office. No gym membership required. No classes to run to after work. You just have to do it at your own pace three times a week.

Body Mass Index Table

	Normal						Overweight					Obese										Extreme Obesity														
BMI	19	20	21	22	23	24	25	26	27	28	29	30	31	32	33	34	35	36	37	38	39	40	41	42	43	44	45	46	47	48	49	50	51	52	53	54
Height (inches)	Body Weight (Pounds)																																			
58	91	96	100	105	110	115	119	124	129	134	138	143	148	153	158	162	167	172	177	181	186	191	196	201	205	210	215	220	224	229	234	239	244	248	253	258
59	94	99	104	109	114	119	124	128	133	138	143	148	153	158	163	168	173	178	183	188	193	198	203	208	212	217	222	227	232	237	242	247	252	257	262	267
60	97	102	107	112	118	123	128	133	138	143	148	153	158	163	168	174	179	184	189	194	199	204	209	215	220	225	230	235	240	245	250	255	261	266	271	276
61	100	106	111	116	122	127	132	137	143	148	153	158	164	169	174	180	185	190	195	201	206	211	217	222	227	232	238	243	248	254	259	264	269	275	280	285
62	104	109	115	120	126	131	136	142	147	153	158	164	169	175	180	186	191	196	202	207	213	218	224	229	235	240	246	251	256	262	267	273	278	284	289	295
63	107	113	118	124	130	135	141	146	152	158	163	169	175	180	186	191	197	203	208	214	220	225	231	237	242	248	254	259	265	270	278	282	287	293	299	304
64	110	116	122	128	134	140	145	151	157	163	169	174	180	186	192	197	204	209	215	221	227	232	238	244	250	256	262	267	273	279	285	291	296	302	308	314
65	114	120	126	132	138	144	150	156	162	168	174	180	186	192	198	204	210	216	222	228	234	240	246	252	258	264	270	276	282	288	294	300	306	312	318	324
66	118	124	130	136	142	148	155	161	167	173	179	186	192	198	204	210	216	223	229	235	241	247	253	260	266	272	278	284	291	297	303	309	315	322	328	334
67	121	127	134	140	146	153	159	166	172	178	185	191	198	204	211	216	223	230	236	242	249	255	261	268	274	280	287	293	299	306	312	319	325	331	338	344
68	125	131	138	144	151	158	164	171	177	184	190	197	203	210	216	223	230	236	243	249	256	262	269	276	282	289	295	302	308	315	322	328	335	341	348	354
69	128	135	142	149	155	162	169	176	182	189	196	203	209	216	223	230	236	243	250	257	263	270	277	284	291	297	304	311	318	324	331	338	345	351	359	365
70	132	139	146	153	160	167	174	181	188	195	202	209	216	222	229	236	243	250	257	264	271	278	285	292	299	306	313	320	327	334	341	348	355	362	369	376
71	136	143	150	157	165	172	179	186	193	200	208	215	222	229	236	243	250	257	265	272	279	286	293	301	308	315	322	329	338	343	351	358	365	372	379	386
72	140	147	154	162	169	177	184	191	199	206	213	221	228	235	242	250	258	265	272	279	287	294	302	309	316	324	331	338	346	353	361	368	375	383	390	397
73	144	151	159	166	174	182	189	197	204	212	219	227	235	242	250	257	265	272	280	288	295	302	310	318	325	333	340	348	355	363	371	378	386	393	401	408
74	148	155	163	171	179	186	194	202	210	218	225	233	241	249	256	264	272	280	287	295	303	311	319	326	334	342	350	358	365	373	381	389	396	404	412	420
75	152	160	168	176	184	192	200	208	216	224	232	240	248	256	264	272	279	287	295	303	311	319	327	335	343	351	359	367	375	383	391	399	407	415	423	431
76	156	164	172	180	189	197	205	213	221	230	238	246	254	263	271	279	287	295	304	312	320	328	336	344	353	361	369	377	385	394	402	410	418	426	435	443

IT'S YOUR BMI THAT MATTERS
WHY BEING A LITTLE FAT IS GOOD—REALLY!

The bathroom scale is a standard tool for anyone trying to get into better shape, but the number it shows isn't the only one you need to pay attention to. You either dread or anticipate what that scale will say, but it's not the be-all and end-all when it comes to weight. It doesn't tell you the whole story. No one would argue that it's a good idea to step on a scale. It's important to keep tabs on your weight, but it's also important to understand what makes up your weight. That's where BMI comes in.

BMI stands for Body Mass Index, which refers to the amount of fat you have. The number is easy to figure out with a calculator: It's your weight in pounds divided by the square root of your height in inches and then multiplied by 703. Your fitness level is then assessed based on where this final number falls on the BMI chart, from underweight to extremely obese.

Your BMI paints a better picture of your health and fitness level than a scale alone. It tells you what you really need to know if you're serious about boosting your metabolism and changing the way you look and feel. For instance, you can reach your goal weight but find that with a high BMI you still don't look the way you want to in a bathing suit. Just because you're lighter doesn't mean you're leaner. If your BMI remains higher than it should be, your metabolism will be slow, and you'll struggle to keep the weight off until you lower your BMI. And more importantly, if your BMI remains high, the greater the risk of developing obesity-related diseases, including heart disease, high blood pressure, stroke, and Type 2 diabetes.

Can you be too lean or fit and fat? Yes! Being too lean is just as unhealthy as being overweight. If your BMI is too low, you are at greater risk for osteoporosis, infertility, malnutrition, thyroid problems, and even hair loss. There is a certain amount of body fat, Essential Body Fat, which is necessary for you to stay healthy. Why? Essential Body Fat helps to regulate metabolism and body temperature, insulate organs, and help with brain functioning, among other things. Fat, contrary to its bad reputation, is actually vital to our survival. It's involved in many important processes—even metabolizing carbohydrates.

Women need more fat than men—that's why they're curvier. The possibility of childbirth creates different hormonal demands on the female body, which affects fat. Men have a different type of fat from women and store it differently.

For basic survival, women need 8 to 12 percent fat, and men require 3 to 5 percent.

Which end of the range you fall into as your optimum depends on your body structure and composition (i.e., are you small, medium, or large-framed?). Your height, whether you build muscle easily, and whether you tend to keep lean muscle more than fat also determine which end of the range you fall into. It should come as no surprise that whether you eat right or work out shows up in your BMI.

Everything else over and above the essential body fat you have is storage fat. And how much excess fat you store depends on your genes, your diet, and on how active you are on a daily basis. *The Metabolism Solution* attacks stored fat more effectively than any other diet plan.

Basically, all fat is made up of three types of fat:

- Visceral Fat. It protects your internal organs but can be very bad for your health if you have too much packed in your abdominal cavity.
- Subcutaneous Fat. Generally the fat you can pinch and the one you most often want to get rid of. Unsightly as it is, it is not as dangerous to you as visceral fat.
- Intramuscular fat. It's interspersed in your muscle tissue. Overtraining or working out the wrong way predisposes you to this type.

Needless to say, you should not aim to get your overall body fat percentage any lower than your essential value—that would be dangerous. It is good to try and keep within your ideal range.

Use the chart on the preceding page or a scale that tells you your BMI. Be consistent with the method you choose and track your BMI weekly. Your BMI will go down if you follow *The Metabolism Solution* as suggested.

I have hundreds, if not thousands, of client stories to pull from where someone tries to explain away why the scale isn't moving or perhaps has even gone in the wrong direction. There's a common theme with many of them: coming home from the gym starved and eating freely. You worked out hard and you've burned calories, so you deserve to eat. That's the reasoning. What it really is, however, is a case of over-exercising.

A LONG WORKOUT COULD LEAD TO A QUICK PIG-OUT.

It seems that lots of people out there are indeed trying to exercise away a bad diet. The media has coined it "Boomeritis" to explain the increase in Baby Boomers ending up in the emergency room from over-exercising. And it's not just Baby Boomers. You can't sit at your desk all week and then let a drill-sergeant-like instructor yell at you and put you through paces meant for an 18-year-old boy. That's

HOME WORKOUTS ARE MORE EFFECTIVE IN LESS TIME.

going to hurt. Now if these militaristic or other methods are working for you, more power to you. But they didn't work for me, and they aren't working for those I counsel every day.

The truth is that over-exercising can make you think you want to eat or, perhaps more accurately, that you deserve to eat. Studies have shown that if you have a hard workout, you may then engage in some "compensatory eating," as it is called. And there goes all your hard work. **You only truly need one third of the calories you consume every day as it is.** Why add even more just because you're exercising? That's counterproductive.

Over-exercising may not only give you a false sense of permission to eat, it may also stress you out. A long workout physically stresses your body—you're breathing hard, sweating, maybe even having shaky limbs. And stress, regardless of whether it's good or bad, produces the same hormone: cortisol. As cortisol levels rise, your body has a propensity to store fat in your midsection and make it easier to gain weight.

Just last year, Columbia University published a study, one of the largest of its kind on exercise and mental health, that found that if you exercise less than 2.5 hours a week you have a higher risk of depression, anxiety, injuries, and overall poor health. Conversely, the study found that exercising more than 7.5 hours a week can make you sick. You read that right. If you're going to the gym two hours a day or stressing over the fact that you can't squeeze it in, stop and keep reading.

METABOLIC EXERCISE VS. EVERYTHING ELSE

All exercise is better than no exercise, but Metabolic Exercise is better than others. You don't have to be a weekend warrior vomiting after a run (which is easier to do than you may think) or a contortionist pulling muscles then not being able to do anything for weeks while you heal. You don't have to be a weightlifter trying to go toe-to-toe with the big boys at the gym and then finding yourself flat on your back with an ice pack and no comfortable position. You do not need to be super-sore to lose weight.

A METABOLIC WORKOUT NOT ONLY BLASTS FAT FASTER, BUT KEEPS BLASTING FAT FOR THE NEXT 36 HOURS.

There is a better way. Metabolic exercise is the most effective way to force your body to burn calories at an accelerated pace, which helps you burn more fat while you exercise. If you google "metabolic exercise" you'll find many plans claiming to offer just that. Don't be fooled.

If your current exercise takes more than 45 minutes a day, it's not metabolic. If you're growing your arms and legs when you're trying to lose inches and tone, it's not metabolic.

If you're dancing for an hour—while it may be fun—it's not metabolic. No dumbbells? It's definitely not metabolic, and it certainly won't strengthen your bones. You may not get the results you want using Pilates, yoga, or Zumba class, either. If you want to burn fat faster, buff up your arms, and slim down your legs, I have good news for you—especially if you are a busy person with barely 10 minutes to spare. A run may be a good idea (if your knees can take it), but a metabolic workout not only blasts fat faster, but keeps blasting fat for the next 36 hours. In 20 to 30 minutes of exercise you can rev up your metabolism for the next day and a half (a thermogenic diet helps). What makes my exercise different? It works every time, as long as you do it.

For your mental and physical health, you absolutely need to move every day. By now you've heard it a thousand times: take the stairs instead of the elevator, park just a little bit further away, walk during your lunch break, and so on. But you only need to do metabolic exercise three times a week—not more. The good news? One workout a week keeps you from backsliding; two workouts will get you results; but three will get you there the fastest. More than that, and it's overkill.

One of the things that stops a fitness plan dead in its tracks is lack of structure and lack of results. If you don't see results in two weeks, stop. When you are on the right track, you know right away if it's working: your clothes start to fit better, you don't ache, and you can do it and keep doing it for the rest of your life. If your routine is too hard, are you going to be able to keep doing it? Are you going to want to? If it's too easy, how long are you going to spend your time with a plan that takes forever to show results?

Let's get back to dumbbells for a moment. If you're on a calorie-reducing diet that does not include strength training, then you are losing muscle. When you increase your muscle, as you do with strength training, you boost your resting metabolic rate—burning more calories even while resting. Lifting weights consumes calories, raises your metabolism, and builds muscles that consume extra calories later on so your body burns more calories even when doing nothing. A 2000 study by G.R. Hunter et al. found that subjects increased their resting metabolic rates after 6 months of resis-

THE BEST SECRET OF ALL: IF YOU EAT RIGHT YOU CAN EXERCISE LESS. The cleaner you eat the less you time you'll need to spend in the gym. You have to learn to eat for what you do. Sitting and watching TV? Guess what: You don't need food. Walking all day shopping? Don't listen to your head hunger: no big meals and definitely no binging required. You need protein, veggies, and carbs that will sustain your activity. Working out? Grab a protein bar or sip a protein shake as you go out the door—or maybe nothing at all. If you eat on my plan, you get exactly what your body needs: no more, no less. And guess what happens when you eat what you need? You begin to burn fat no matter how slow your metabolism is.

tance training and were burning an extra 100 calories a day. Cardio workouts also boost metabolism. In another study, this one by J.A. Potteiger et al., participants did moderate intensity cardio exercise 3 to 5 days per week, 20 to 45 minutes at a time, for 16 months. These subjects increased their resting metabolic rate by burning an extra 129 calories a day. Imagine how walking every day will affect your body. I love the idea of burning an extra 100 calories a day while doing nothing, don't you?

The idea of "more isn't better, better is better" applies to fitness and supplements more than you know, and the reason no one talks about it is that they usually want to sell you something. This is true whether it's a gym membership, expensive bulky equipment, or a trainer who wants you to depend on her while charging you more than you'd care to pay. These may not keep you lean. The secret to living lean and not just getting lean is that whatever gets you fitter and causes you to lose weight is also what keeps those pounds off. Exercise needs to fit into your life, not become your life.

I live in the real world. I'm a wife and mother and work crazy hours every week. I need the fastest, most effective workout that benefits me in the least amount of time. I'm betting that's what you need, too. Who has three or six hours a day to spend in the gym? Not me. That's why your diet needs to support your results.

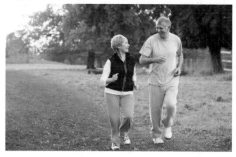

THE STARTING LINE

Most people have no clue where to begin when it comes to an exercise program. Starting is simpler than you think. Exercise is about more than weight loss; it's about making you stronger, more flexible, and in cardiovascular shape. When you exercise, all kinds of miraculous things happen. Your immune system is stimulated; you're energized and detoxified; depression lifts; your skin gets tighter (especially if you're eating right); your bone density improves; and perhaps best of all, aging is not only slowed but reversed. You can't make excuses when all this and more is on the line.

I always have new clients take a fitness test, one that I've developed over the years. Not only do I assess their physical ability, but I ask hard questions about their goals, activity, and mindset. You need to assess in order to know what you need to do and what you need to change to get there. I have my clients walk for 20 minutes, check their BMI score, do pushups and planks, and I check their flexibility. I ask them questions—like those in The Slow Metabolism Test—about their general health.

READY, SET, GO! THE 1-MILE WALK TEST

Get your walking shoes out. This test measures your aerobic (cardiovascular) fitness level based on how quickly you can walk one mile at moderate intensity. Warm up by walking slowly for a few minutes and when you are ready to begin, start the clock. At the end be sure to follow up with some stretches. Please don't try this unless you are regularly walking for 15 to 20 minutes several times a week. Times given in minutes and seconds. These standards are based on information from the American College of Sports Medicine (acsm.org).

Age	20-29	30-39	40-49	50-59	60-69	70+
Women						
Excellent	< 13:12	< 12:24	< 12:54	< 12:24	< 14:06	< 15:06
Good	11:54-13:00	12:24-13:30	12:54-14:00	13:24-14:24	14:06-15:12	15:06-15:48
Average	13:01-14:30	13:31-14:12	14:01-14:42	14:25-15:12	15:13-16:18	15:49-18:48
Fair	13:43-14:30	14:13-15:00	14:43-15:30	15:13-16:30	16:19-17:18	18:49-20:18
Poor	> 14:30	> 15:00	>15:30	> 16:30	> 17:18	>20:18
Men						
Excellent	< 13.12	< 13:42	< 14:12	< 14:42	< 15:06	< 18:18
Good	13:12-14:06	13:42-14:36	14:12-15:06	14:42-15:36	15:06-16:18	18:18-20:00
Average	14:07-15:06	14:37-15:36	15:07-16:06	15:37-17:00	16:19-17:30	20:01-21:48
Fair	15:07-16:30	15:37-17:-00	16:07-17:30	17:01-18:06	17:31-19:12	21:49-24:06
Poor	> 16.30	> 17:00	> 17.30	> 18.06	> 19.12	> 24.06

THE ONE-MINUTE PUSHUP TEST

A pushup is the best way to determine your overall fitness—especially your upper body strength. Set a timer and go. Men use a traditional pushup position; women can start on knees if needed. No clapping between pushups required. (Developed by the American College of Sports Medicine, acsm.org)

Women	Age 20-29	30-39	40-49	50-59	60-69
Excellent	30	27	24	21	17
Very Good	21-29	20-26	12-23	11-20	12-16
Good	15-20	13-19	11-14	7-10	5-11
Fair	10-14	8-12	5-10	2-6	2-4
Needs Improvement	9	7	4	1	1

Men	Age 20-29	30-39	40-49	50-59	60-69
Excellent	36	30	25	21	18
Very Good	29-35	22-29	17-24	13-20	11-17
Good	22-28	17-21	13-16	10-12	8-10
Fair	17-21	12-16	10-12	7-9	5-7
Needs Improvement	16	11	9	6	4

If all you are looking to do is just work out, there are so many options: P90X, Insanity, Cross Fit, Zumba, and more. If you want more flexibility, then Pilates and yoga may be calling to you. But if you are looking to lose weight because your metabolism needs a kick-start (and you'll know if you take The Slow Metabolism Test), it's time for a change. It's not you who has failed; your fitness program has failed you.

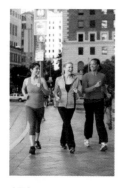

THE METABOLIC CORE WALK

The first step, no pun intended, of a metabolic workout is the Metabolic Core Walk. Done daily, it strengthens your bones and heart and boosts your metabolism. The Metabolic Core Walk, a cardio workout, is the most important step in boosting your metabolism. If you did nothing but this walk for 45 to 60 minutes daily, you would change your body shape fast.

So what is it? Metabolic Core Walking is walking with good posture at a speed that revs up the calorie burn. That's not a casual stroll while window shopping, and it's not a jog either. You should feel like you're gliding, not pounding the pavement. Walk forward gently as if you're pushing a carriage. The next time you're at the market, get a feel for it when pushing your shopping cart down the aisles. It's walking with a sense of urgency, back straight, arms moving. Walk with your core—as if you're squeezing a golf ball in your buttocks and keeping your stomach muscles pulled in tight. Just don't confuse good posture with tensing your shoulders and raising them to your ears. Imagine God is pulling a string coming from your chest, so you keep your neck nice and long and your shoulders back and down.

> **WHEN METABOLIC CORE WALKING, IMAGINE GOD IS PULLING A STRING FROM YOUR CHEST SO YOU KEEP YOUR NECK LONG AND YOUR SHOULDERS BACK AND DOWN.**

THE PLANK TEST: CORE STRENGTH AND ENDURANCE

How strong is your core? A strong core keeps you free from injury and your back in tip-top shape for the rest of your life. If your core isn't strong enough, you're not fit enough. The Plank Test is not only a way to gauge your core's fitness; it's also what you need to do to get your core strong. Doing a plank two to three times a week (with one day between each), you can get fit fast. Find an exercise mat or a comfortable spot on the floor and assume a pushup position but with your weight on your forearms instead of your hands. Contract your stomach muscles as if you're about to be punched. Now hold it. Your body should form a straight line from shoulders to ankles.

If you can't make it for one minute, you need to work on your core strength. The remedy is planks two to three times a week for as long as you can until you build up endurance. Over two minutes? You are strong.

Start with 20 minutes a day until you can walk 5 miles in 60 minutes; you want to be able to walk a 12- to 15-minute mile without feeling like you're having a heart attack. And you don't have to do it all in one stretch. You can break it up, say, into 20-minute increments. That's it. Walking. Your knees will thank you, and so will the rest of you. And you can walk anywhere, anytime. There's no need to ever step foot in a gym.

If it's pouring rain or snowing, I take it inside. Treadmills are great to keep you walking, whatever the weather, and even better at keeping you at a consistent speed. Those times when I'm having an off day (I get them, too), I jump on my stationary bike and ride more than an hour at a lower tension. (Many drafts of this book were read and edited while I pedaled away.) The bike really helps if you can't walk due to injury but can still pedal. It's crucial that you continue exercising in some capacity. I'm not a fan of outdoor bikes for fat loss. Aside from weather factoring in whether you work out or not, you can't keep a consistent speed (because of the hills on the road and obstacles like cars and people) on an outdoor bike. Think of investing in a treadmill or stationary bike. With one, you can absolutely never use the excuse of "I couldn't walk/ride today; it was too rainy."

DUMBBELLS FOR SMART WORKOUTS

Before you think it's inevitable that you'll end up with frail bones as you get older, consider that working out with weights in your hands at least twice a week strengthens your bones. Pilates, yoga, and dancing don't do that as effectively or efficiently. Twenty minutes a week can halt osteoporosis. Your bones need you to work out with weights. What are you waiting for? You don't need to spend $2,000 on some fancy machine with adjustable pulleys and cables. You don't need to join a gym. Dumbbells, hand weights—any brand that you can hold comfortably and purchase in your local discount store—will do. Even a can will do in a pinch.

YOUR BONES NEED YOU TO WORK OUT WITH WEIGHTS!

Dumbbells have never gone out of fashion with those serious about fitness. The moves shown on the following pages will boost your metabolism. A metabolic workout may be quick compared to some workouts, but it is highly effective. It shouldn't kill you, but if it feels easy, you're not doing it right. Go deeper, squeeze harder and tighter. Add another set of reps or use heavier weights. Keep going. Each move combines three of your major muscle groups with minimal rest between. You will sweat, but you won't be left shaky and pale on the floor. Just because these exercises are good for your metabolism does not mean more exercise is better. Three times a week. Stick to the plan. (Note: if you can hold the weights in your hands as per the pictures, great! If not, you can perform the move without the weights.)

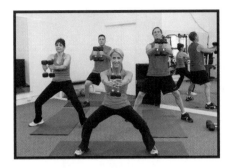

The 30-Minute Metabolic Workout

1. Deep Squat to Front Raise. Stand with feet shoulder width apart with dumbbells in hands in front. Squat down and stand back up, raising dumbbells to chin level.

2. Stiff Leg Dead Lift. Stand with legs together, knees slightly bent, dumbbells in hands. Bend at waist, lowering weights to the ground, using the back of the leg bring them back up to knee level.

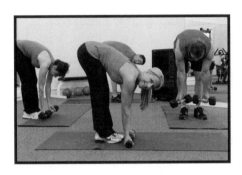

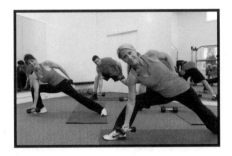

3. Side Lunge with Arm Curl. Lunge to side with weight in hand. Lower weight to lunging leg, pushing with your heel back to start position, while simultaneously bringing dumbbell to your waist in a curl.

4. Front Lunge with Side Raise. Holding dumbbells in hand, step or lunge forward to front lunge position; perform side dumbbell raises. Or perform side dumbbell raises in a front lunge position (you decide which is best).

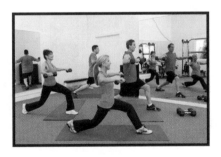

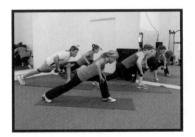

5. Bent Over Dumbbell Row in Lunge Position. Holding dumbbells in hand, bend over from the waist while in front lunge position; perform dumbbell rows by lowering weights to the floor and pulling them back up (as if starting a lawn mower).

6. Tricep Dip. Place hands at the edge of your seat and lower your body to the floor, using your arms to raise yourself back up. Be sure to keep your body close to seat/chair and squeeze your arms at the top of the move.

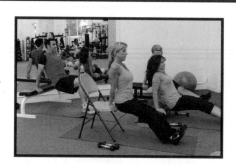

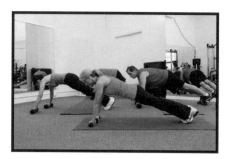

7. Pushups. Lay down face first on floor and hands next to chest. Push yourself up until body is parallel with floor. Keep your body straight and core tight.

8. Lying Rear Fly. Lying face down with dumbbells in hands out to side. Raise dumbbells back as if you were "reverse flying."

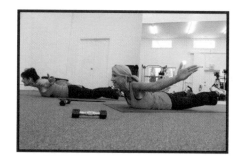

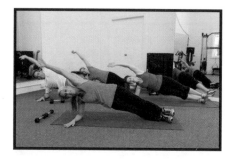

9. Side Core Raise. Lying on your side on your elbow, lift your body off floor using your core. Too hard? Use an arm or leg to help at first.

10. Plank. Lie face first on floor, body straight. Come up on elbows and toes using abs to lift. Hold as long as you can, aiming for 1 minute.

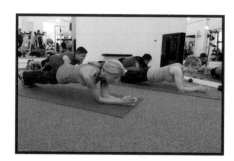

POSTURE POWER

They say the camera adds 10 pounds to your appearance. Proper posture takes those pounds away. Try it. When you stand your straightest, you pull in your gut and use muscles you wouldn't be using otherwise. You look slimmer—but you're also burning more calories, strengthening your muscles, and breathing better.

When was the last time you heard someone tell you to stand up straight? To stop slouching in your chair? Poor posture is to blame for most back and neck pain—not to mention chronic joint pain. Posture is something you don't hear much about, but good posture is one of the most under-utilized solutions that can change everything for you.

GOT BACK PAIN? A WEAK CORE IS TO BLAME.

I have seen more people get in shape only to not look any better or different because they worked out with bad posture and only made it worse. Did you know that the average person overworks biceps, abs, and legs in workouts? These muscles pull you forward, while the butt, hamstrings, triceps, and back keep you straight. Strengthening these muscles is the key to correcting the slumped posture that brings on pain.

Just about every client I know who experiences back and neck pain usually tucks her pelvis and tightens her glutes (butt), hyper-extends her knees, turns out her feet, rounds the upper back, and sticks out her neck. Maybe you do all of these things, and most overweight people do all of them because their bodies adapt to carrying the load. But just because a body adapts does not mean it's a good idea. So what's so bad about doing this?

Butt tucking, also known as tucking your pelvis under, puts your whole body out of alignment and causes sway back, making your butt look flat and sloping your shoulders. This creates a domino effect from your head to your toes: Tucking your pel-

THE TOE TOUCH TEST

No other test is so easy or so telling. Can you touch your toes? If you can touch them, you will be about **300 percent less likely to lose your** posture or have posture issues. Posture is everything when it comes to keeping your body healthy.

Do the test: Put your feet together, bend over, and reach for your toes. Your knees need to be kept straight. Can you touch your toes with straight knees? If you can, you pass; if not, you need to work on strengthening your core muscles and your flexibility. Follow the balanced workouts and stretches in this book to correct imbalances; other programs may actually cause muscle imbalances by overworking some muscles while not working others hard enough. A fit body is a healthy body.

If you cannot reach your toes, you risk suffering from loss of spine posture—and the health of your spine determines the health of your body. That's why doctors have you bend over and touch your toes in a routine physical. With that one test, they can check your hamstrings, glutes, abs, and hip mobility. A failed toe touch can lead to back problems, and it lets you know you need the Recovery Stretch.

183

vis forces your feet and legs to rotate out, which in turn triggers low back and hip pain. This type of slouch also puts more pressure on your feet than they can handle, as they are not designed to carry the load, potentially leading to flat feet and/or plantar fasciitis. But hold on, it doesn't stop there.

When feet are not aligned, your knees take a beating, and your tucked pelvis flattens the lumbar spine, removing the natural curve of the lower back. We need this natural curve for balance so we don't fall backwards. This is why we round our backs forward and stick our necks out—it's our body's way of adjusting so we don't fall backwards.

LOOK LEANER

You can stand straighter. Get in front of a mirror and stand like this: Start off as if God has a string attached to the top of your chest and is lifting you up—this is better for posture than a string to your head.

Take a deep breath and exhale hard, releasing all the stress you're holding in your body.

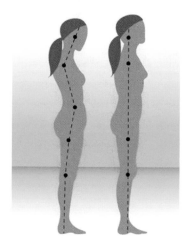

1. Relax your shoulders and keep them pushed down and back.
2. Be sure your ears, shoulders and hips, knees, and ankles all line up vertically.
3. Pull your chin back so your head isn't out in front (this helps get rid of turkey neck).
4. Keep your pelvis neutral or arched back (vs. tucked under), glutes relaxed. Remember, you want a straight line.
5. Feet should be hip-distance apart and toes facing forward.

That's your starting point. Don't worry if you're feeling overwhelmed; it may very well be a sign that you need this big time if normal posture feels so hard to you. Remember that imaginary golf ball? I always tell my clients to squeeze that imaginary golf ball—in the glutes for men, the pelvic floor (like Kegel exercises) for women. This really helps teach your body's core (abs) how to do its job. Any time you feel back pain, pull in your stomach, go through the quick and easy steps listed above, and it may just disappear.

Sitting posture is the same, except your legs should not be crossed and you need to get up every 20 minutes and move or your discs slam together and cement in place. Not good. That's why drinking lots of water helps pain and lubricates your joints so they glide easily. This will also insure that you get up every 20 minutes—you'll have to pee and that's a good thing on both counts. Also, be sure to have the right seat. I like a stool that I straddle so I sit actively and do not slump. If your chair allows you to slump, get rid of it and sit on a bar stool; you'll have less back pain because your core is working, (that's its job), not your joints. The core has incredible endurance, when strengthened and used, and will protect your joints.

Old habits die hard, so if you are a leg crosser like me, switch legs every hour when you sit. Also switch if you tend to stand on one leg (put all your weight on one side). Standing with one leg supporting most of your weight throws your pelvis out of alignment and leaves you unbalanced.

> **STAND TALL: YOU'LL STRENGTHEN YOUR MUSCLES, BREATHE BETTER, AND BURN MORE CALORIES.**

STRETCHING TO THE HEAVENS

Remember the old childhood song "Head, Shoulders, Knees, and Toes" and how you'd touch each body part as you sang? Can you still do that? Can you touch your toes? If you want better moving muscles, you have to stretch—and not just the kind you do when you have a big yawn. As you age, your muscles tighten and movement can become painful. Stretching helps increase the range of motion of your joints and improve your flexibility. It improves your posture and gives you better blood flow. Daily stretching is the secret to reducing soreness and tightness so you can keep walking and doing your metabolic workout. You'll find the more comprehensive Recovery Stretch on my DVD, but Lazy Man's Yoga works in a pinch.

I developed it after helping countless people who turned to me for workouts after injuring themselves through either over-exercise or other means. All my moves are done lying on your back using your core muscles to keep your body grounded on the floor. Breathing is very important to stretching, and it's vital that you exhale often. Breathing changes everything when it comes to stretching; it sends messages to your muscles that they should relax and let go of stress.

Not only will stretching give you better-looking muscles, but it can also help with joint pain as well. Pain, no matter what the cause or your age, is your body's way of letting you know that it's out of balance. Pain is a symptom that something is wrong; it's an alarm saying, "De-stress, relax." Your body is telling you that you need to move. I always tell my clients, "If you rest, you'll rust." Exercise keeps your body limber and increases circulation all over, which delivers the nutrients your body needs to heal. Exercise also removes toxins, making it critical when it comes to keeping your body in working order so that you feel good. And I know from my own personal experience that when I feel good, I eat better.

Remember, you can always stretch on those days when you're not feeling very well. Our joints are designed like bladders, and they need to be emptied in order to feel better. Have you ever noticed that you always feel better when you exercise, and your aches and pains go away? There really is no excuse not to exercise. If you're short on time, do 15 minutes of the DVD in the morning and the other 15 after work.

Tight muscles are a symptom of an over-stressed body that could be prone to injury. Best way to avoid this? Stretch. The wear and tear of obsessive exercising, doing the wrong exercise, or doing the right exercise the wrong way can be alleviated by stretching. After all, workouts are supposed to make you feel better, not worse. Stress less, eat less.

Lazy Man's Yoga

Don't forget to breathe!

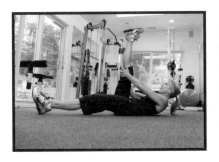

1. The Back Fixer (Lying 90-Degree Stretch). Lie flat on your back and bring your leg straight to 90 degrees. Repeat other side.

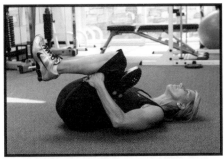

4. The Butt Stretch/Hip Opener. On back, bend leg at 90-degree angle and place ankle of opposite foot in front of knee; then pull knee back to feel stretch in butt and hips. Repeat other side.

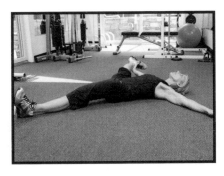

2. Lying Inner Thigh Stretch. Lie flat on back and stretch leg as far away from body as possible. Keep leg as straight as possible. Repeat other side.

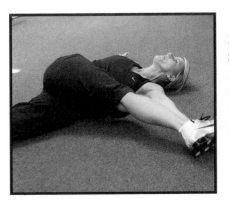

3. Lying Outer Thigh Stretch. Lie flat on back and bring leg over and across your body (right leg crosses over left and out to left side). Keep leg as straight as possible.

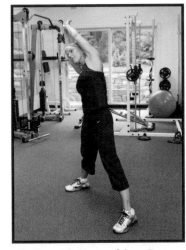

5. Stretch Everything Out Stretch. Catch your breath. Raise arms above head and gently lean to each side, holding stretch 8 to 10 seconds.

SIX

METABOLISM MIND GAMES

One of my favorite sayings is, "Where your head goes, your body follows." I believe your thoughts determine your outcomes because they guide you, powering your decisions right from the start. Your thoughts point you in certain directions that ultimately determine your end results, create your attitudes and perspectives, and affect your relationships—specifically with your own body. Your thoughts determine how productive both the weight loss and the transformation will be, and they influence every decision you need to make.

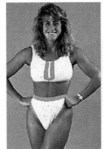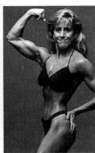

Transformation happens when you believe it can happen!

I realize looking back at my own background, during my time participating and helping in Dr. Hatfield's study, that I wasn't successful at losing weight because deep down I really didn't believe it was going to happen for me. I never even tried to do what needed to be done, complaining that a certain diet didn't work for me or a particular workout didn't give me the results I wanted because it wouldn't. I believed what I was telling myself (I couldn't change), and my body simply agreed with me by staying fat. And even when I saw some transformation, I couldn't believe it because I was so buried in negative feelings about my body.

I struggled, hated my body, and wanted to change it so badly I could taste it. While crying about how miserable I was, I continued to eat all the wrong foods—the foods that were keeping me fat and slowing down my metabolism. I would exercise on and off, some days like a fiend, others not at all. And when it came to keeping a food and exercise journal, as we were all required to do for the study, I told myself and the other participants I was eating perfectly and exercising.

I truly believed I was eating healthy and exercising correctly. This is known as a sincere lie: you believe what you tell yourself, regardless of its actual validity. For the study, I would literally sit in front of Dr. Hatfield's office and fill in my food/exercise journal with what he wanted to see, what he expected me to do. When weigh-in time came, anxiety would set in, and I would find myself coming up with any and every excuse as to why the scale didn't budge. It was stress; it was my period; of course I was following the plan and couldn't imagine why I wasn't losing weight. Sound a little familiar? I cannot believe I did that. It seems comical now, but it sure wasn't at the time.

Why tell you this embarrassing story? Because every day I get thousands of emails saying something very similar: "I'm doing everything right, and I'm still not losing." My first response is to ask for a glimpse of this "perfect" food journal. The food journal reveals all; often it's filled with foods that slow the metabolism and cause weight gain—even the so-called healthy ones. There's bacon, whole eggs, whole-grain, organic bread, gluten-free pasta, avocados, nuts, yogurt, and cheese. Often I see a whey protein shake made with fruit, juice, and soy, almond, rice, or even cow's milk. Not helpful if you are trying to lose weight. Others add a whey protein shake to an already fattening and carbohydrate-filled breakfast instead of having just the shake for breakfast, as intended. No wonder the calories add up.

Then there's the complaint that they are doing Pilates/yoga/(insert your favorite workout) all the time and not seeing results. *The Metabolism Solution* is specific in which metabolic exercises to do. Doing an hour on the StairMaster and then coming home from the gym famished is overworking. Do you have two or more hours a day to exercise? I don't.

We are human and far from perfect. It can be hard to stick to a food plan and hard to fit in the exercise. *The Metabolism Solution* takes this into account. Forgive yourself for not being perfect. No one is. *The Metabolism Solution* is guaranteed to work every time if you follow the plan and eat accordingly. It is so effective—and here's a little secret I probably shouldn't tell you—that you will lose weight even if you do not exercise. Do not let "I don't have time to exercise" be your mantra. Don't get stuck thinking only about what you cannot do—think about what you can do. Miracles happen in I cans.

TURNING NEGATIVITY INTO POSSIBILITY

Do you think you're a glass-half-full or glass-half-empty kind of person? Do you let past mistakes drive you? Do you forever see yourself as the label with which an abusive person branded you? Perhaps an early childhood experience has scarred you and influenced you in more ways than you realize. Have you ever asked yourself what your weight gain represents? The answer may surprise you.

STAND TALL: YOU'LL STRENGTHEN YOUR MUSCLES, BREATHE BETTER, AND BURN MORE CALORIES.

You have to choose to put the past behind you and move forward. I come from a divorced household with two alcoholic parents. If there were a Dysfunctional Family Olympics, we could have won the gold medal. I get how hurt feels; it is so hard to find faith and acceptance when bad things happen, but it's a choice you need to make. You have to trade your negative attitude for a positive one and believe you can be happy and healthy. But you have to decide to do so first. Dwelling on the pain keeps you in pain. When you complain, you'll remain.

If you can move on from it, you can change your life. You don't need to be angry to heal, and you don't resolve resentments with anger. Anger keeps you stuck where you are. Same unfulfilling job, same un-appreciative spouse, same number on the scale. It's so easy to feed anger and resentment. You eat to ease the pain, then you gain weight and that causes more pain. So you eat again. Your initial solution to pain is now the problem.

A key, perhaps, is to live in the present, to feel gratitude for every God-given day, to feel hope that to-morrow is a new chance to try again. Once you have set your mind to let go of anger and resentment, stick to it and say the words of possibility every day: I Can. Start right now; turn your negativity into possibility. It isn't easy, so fake it until you make it—it works if you work at it. Don't keep repeating, "It will never happen for me." It is up to you. There are no excuses. Start now: Put all of your energy into the doing, and you'll get results faster than you ever have before. Discipline comes from the do-ing, and motivation follows.

Letting go of anger and resentment removes the num-ber one obstacle in the way of you leading the life God has in store for you. If you believe, you will achieve; and where there is a will, there is always a way. Stop using and believing in the words I can't. Working with other professional trainers and celebrities like Martha Stewart has taught me that we all wake up with the same amount of time in a day, and we all have the same choices. It's simply a question of whether we will make the right choices. With the information found here on weight loss and how to exercise effectively, nothing is

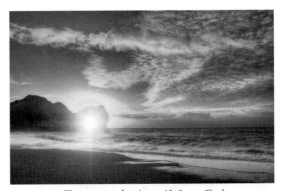

Every new day is a gift from God

standing in your way. Take it one day at a time, one meal at a time, one workout at a time. You cannot take a day "off" while trying to lose weight because it will stop your momentum and slow your me-tabolism. You don't need to trigger bad eating that isn't helpful in the long run. Change your thoughts, and you'll change your body. Quitting is not an option because failure is not an option. This has worked for me for over 25 years.

It also helps me to stay positive by surrounding myself with positive people. I had the self-pity parties that would paralyze me and stop me from making the changes needed to get control of my weight. Misery loves company, and you can always find those (the overeaters and under-exercisers) who will agree with you and support your negativity. Change isn't necessarily easy; surround yourself with people who have the same goals as you do so you can inspire and support each other. Find those who think it and do it. Find that ability in each other.

You don't need more people around you to help you eat the wrong things or keep you from the gym. It's time to find a workout buddy and see if your friends will eat healthy and forego desserts with you. Look around and think out of the box here; the best partners may be the least obvious. Family members often mean well, but they are often the ones to teach us wrong eating and negative thinking.

Look for people at work or others who have the same goal in mind and create a relationship of accountability where you each let the other know when you need help getting back on track with your food or exercise. Allow them to be firm in order to get you back on track by not letting you give any excuses. There isn't any reason why you shouldn't be taking care of your body by eating right and exercising. Eating clean, as with *The Metabolism Solution*, and exercising are the solution to almost every problem—from weight loss to achy joints to fibromyalgia to injuries to depression. No matter the issue, you cannot go wrong with exercise, eating your veggies, and lean protein.

EMOTIONAL EATING 101

Emotional eaters eat when they are happy, or sad, or even when bored. How do you know if you are an emotional eater? You know. Trust me. When I meet a new client, red flags immediately go up if he asks me during that very first session about eating a certain food or if he'll be able to go "off" the plan. Such questions tell me right away that this is someone looking for an excuse to cheat before he even begins. This is no judgment from me; it takes one to know one, and I am one of these people. Experience has taught me that a different approach and attitude makes all the difference. "I'll do whatever it takes," and "I'll do it as long as it takes" are the words and thoughts to live by when striving for weight loss. Do you need that glass or two of wine every day? Or to treat yourself with food? If you're saying yes, then this is an indication that you use food to avoid feelings, or at least the uncomfortable ones. Those that answer no treat themselves to manicures, a movie, or new clothes—not a food reward. We're rewarded with food from childhood. (Ice cream after the school concert?) But this is a sure way to get fat and not the way to lose weight.

Those people who don't think of food as a comfort, who don't self-medicate with it, don't eat when stressed. They actually often forget to eat. If you look to food to make yourself feel better, you eat more.

> **YOUR ATTITUDE DETERMINES YOUR ALTITUDE**
>
> How do we become compulsive overeaters who can't stop? How do we get our food under control? All behavior arises from a state of stress. Between the behavior and the stress is a primary emotion. Remember that there are only two primary emotions, love and fear.
>
> It is through the expression or processing (also known as feeling) and the understanding of the fear that we can calm the stress and dismiss the behavior.

Food addicts are emotional eaters. They live for food and think about it all day long compared to non-addicts, who need to remember to eat and don't spend the day thinking about their next "hit," as if food were a drug. Unfortunately, that is a perfect way to think of food—as a drug. Studies show that food, especially sugar, hits the same spot in our brain as drugs, hooking us and making us dependent on the very foods we should be avoiding. With a food addiction, you can never have just one of anything; the whole bag disappears in the blink of an eye. Then what happens? You want more of that treat (potato chips, Yodels, doughnuts, bread—you name it) and will find yourself stocking up at the store and eating it every night.

It was not easy for me to get past this. I got "clean" with food by following a 12-step program. Over-eaters Anonymous is a 12-step program that has the highest success rate in helping emotional eaters and food addicts. It taught me that compulsive overeating is a three-fold disease: 1) Physical, sometimes you are just hardwired to want to eat more; 2) Mental, you are prone to short-circuit during times of stress; and 3) Spiritual, if you're not in a good relationship with God, you will struggle.

Nothing else that you might find on the Internet or in a bookstore will help. All the information out there can paralyze you with misinformation. It will have you thinking you can't when you should be empowered by the information right here on these pages and ready to take control of your life.

YOUR RELATIONSHIP WITH YOURSELF DETERMINES YOUR OUTCOME

Your success rides completely on where your head is at, so to speak. If you are a positive person who thinks positively, you will get positive results. Have faith in yourself and in God. But what if you are more like me and struggle with depression and self-doubt? It's not so easy to turn a negative attitude into a positive one when you feel so awful.

To help turn the tide, you need to do these three things every day:

1. Exercise. Exercise helps release happy hormones, and we can never get enough of these.
2. Drink your shake daily. The right kind of whey protein provides the mood boost and nutrients needed to get your brain working at its best.
3. Supplement safely. Safe supplements replace lost nutrients that anxiety siphons from our bodies at an accelerated pace, creating the need for more.

I know exactly what you are thinking and where you are coming from. I have been there. Just remember that you have nothing to lose except weight, and if you try it and don't feel better, I'll refund your misery.

The proverbial light bulb turned on over my head when I was working with Bryan Post, one of the nation's leading child behavior experts. I learned that instead of feeling an emotion, I eat. I'd rather eat than let myself be stressed, mad, or angry. What I have had to learn and accept—and perhaps you do, too—is that all emotions are valid and should be felt. Emotions are simply emotions. It's not normal to be numb, or to feel nothing; when we overeat, we numb ourselves from pain, fear, anger, and more. Unfortunately, when we block these negative emotions, we block the positive ones as well. Husbands, kids, parents, and even pets avoid us unless we approach them from a peaceful, loving place. Have you ever noticed that? You push away the very things you want so desperately by stifling all emotions.

> **WOULD YOU RATHER EAT THAN LET YOURSELF BE STRESSED, MAD, OR ANGRY?**

When you are "food sober" you allow yourself to feel all feelings, work them through, and let them be. So when you are feeling stressed or upset, stop and think a moment before you open the refrigerator. Food is the problem, not the solution, and it's keeping you from feeling the required feelings you are supposed to experience.

Using an addictive behavior to deal with stress is far too common. Shopping and even compulsive exercise are all "drugs" that can become just as addictive as food or alcohol. Eating is a way of running away from uncomfortable feelings. You can run, but you cannot hide, from these uncomfortable emotions. They have a way of hunting you down—sometimes when you least expect it. It's not always easy, but it's best to look that fear in the eye and tell it that you are not afraid. You are on your side. I am on your side. Most of all, God is on your side. And for me, knowing that God is on *my* side has turned out to be all I need.

So how is your relationship with yourself? Not so good? Are you convinced you will love yourself if you just get a flat stomach, lean legs, or stop eating like a glutton? Real, lasting change occurs when we love ourselves. We have to love ourselves *first*.

HEAD HUNGER GAMES

Typically, there are two things that motivate people to do what needs to be done to change: love and fear. When you act out of a place of love for yourself, you tend to want to eat healthfully; you exercise to nurture your body and to keep it in working order. You do the right thing, and not because you are afraid. Fear derails you. Fear makes you stressed and anxious, and these two factors are the number one cause of overeating and bingeing. They are the reasons your hunger switch doesn't turn off.

Think about it for a second. Are you 25 pounds overweight? You know you are supposed to eat more vegetables, aiming for 10 servings and a little protein four times a day. Yet instead, you think you're hungry and grab a crunchy snack or a sugar-filled food. Is your body physically hungry? Probably not. This is head hunger. And feeding this head hunger is what hurts the most.

Just as you reboot your metabolism, you can reboot how you react to your body's hunger signals and learn to eat when truly, physically hungry and stop when full. The Halt Principle is a simple test. Before you reach for that midmorning doughnut, HALT. Ask yourself:

Am I **H**ungry?
Am I **A**ngry or **A**nxious?
Am I **L**onely?
Am I **T**ired?

Simple questions, right? Wrong. These are loaded questions, but it is totally possible to change your not-so-favorable habits into ones that boost your metabolism. How? Well, you can't avoid stress, but you can change how you deal with it. Stress hormones can add to belly fat, but did you know that stress can also help you lose weight at a faster rate? It's true.

We all know someone who has been under stress and seems to waste away, but eating because we are stressed is the true culprit when it comes to weight gain. Eating certain foods like crunchy carbs, yummy sweets, sauce-drenched staples (like the popular comfort food macaroni and cheese) adds fat fast. When you add fat-filled food to your diet, your fat cells take it as a signal to store fat. On the other hand, eating lean and clean proteins and vegetables does not cause fat to be stored under stressful conditions.

Sometimes, you might find yourself feeling hungry all the time. Even after eating. If you are following *The Metabolism Solution*, you are eating enough to fill your body's gas tank. You will not starve, I promise you. This is head hunger taunting you. Being hungry is a good sign when on my plan; it means your metabolism is moving, and you are burning fat. Don't give in.

If you are serious about losing weight and living a leaner lifestyle, this is what you need to do: Wait at least five minutes before eating when you are under stress and think you are hungry. Hit the pause button and wait. Pray. You will make better choices by not trying to feed the stress to make it go away, and you won't be adding to your stress because you feel guilty about what you ate.

If someone had told me that my anxiety and fear were making me overeat, I could have spared myself 20 years of self-loathing and wrecked vacations. Looking back, I see now that I hated my

> WHEN YOU'RE STRESSED AND REACHING FOR THAT SUGARY SNACK, HIT THE PAUSE BUTTON. YOU WILL MAKE BETTER CHOICES BY NOT TRYING TO FEED THE STRESS TO MAKE IT GO AWAY, AND YOU WON'T BE ADDING TO YOUR STRESS BECAUSE YOU FEEL GUILTY ABOUT WHAT YOU ATE.

body so much I never enjoyed anything—not swimming and especially not shopping. I never bought any new clothes because I was waiting until I reached that magic number on the scale. And once I reached my goal weight, I still did not get rid of my fat clothes because I didn't believe I could keep the weight off; I had too-good-to-be-true syndrome and was waiting for the other shoe to drop. This kind of stinking thinking is always present when you don't love yourself. When you love yourself, you want to take better care of your body.

If you are serious about real results and permanent change, are you doing what needs to be done? Are you willing to do it? Can you change your thinking?

Change your thoughts, and they become actions. What you think about is what you focus on and repeatedly do; if you think positively, you will find yourself with positive action. Thinking negatively will stop you from staying on the plan, which works if you stay on it. Positive thinking can bring you peace—and that is always a good outcome. Surrender fully to the process. One hundred percent.

> BY REPEATEDLY WRITING DOWN YOUR GOAL, YOU CAN ENGRAVE IT INTO YOUR SUBCONSCIOUS— "BRAINWASHING" YOURSELF.

Set your mind and keep it set; do not fall into self-sabotaging analysis. There is so much misinformation available. Log off your computer, close the books, and focus on the fast results you will see when following *The Metabolism Solution*. It works 100 percent of the time if you do it.

Practice good habits daily and do not quit. Quitting is not an option and should not even be in your vocabulary anymore. Practice until you arrive at your dream weight and, once you arrive, you can decide then whether you choose to eat more freely—but you may find that it's just not worth it anymore because food has lost its power over you. Yes, it does happen.

> PERFECTION DOES **NOT** EXIST.
> 80 PERCENT IS AS PERFECT AS IT GETS. FOCUS ON PROGRESS INSTEAD.

Turn your fear into faith. Stop worrying and doubting and just do it. Any training and any small eating change is better than no change at all.

Fake it until you make it. When you wake up feeling defeated, you will fake it until you are over the negative thoughts. Repeat after me, "I am doing this. I can do this. I'm a lean, mean, fighting machine. I love me." My daily mantra was Leaner, Stronger. I repeated this over and over the entire time I was on the treadmill for 60 minutes a day, and I also wrote it down 100 times every night.

Focus on progress, not perfection. Perfection does not exist and you will fall down, so learn to forgive yourself. You now love yourself—remember?—and we forgive people we love, including ourselves. Eighty percent is as perfect as it gets. Learn to love yourself no matter what. This is your primary goal.

Let go and let God. I believe in a higher power, and that higher power for me is God. He has you in the palm of His hand, always.

This cycle of eating because we feel bad and then feeling bad because we've eaten is a very slippery slope and can easily spiral out of control. This is why we gain weight and continue to gain weight until we finally are sick and tired of being sick and tired.

How can you handle cravings? A craving can be crushed by distracting yourself. Change your thought, move a muscle. Exercise is the best remedy. I need to keep busy to stop myself from thinking about food all day long. Now that I am thinking lean, I turn to my list of to-do's before I open the refrigerator if I think I'm hungry after a meal. It has helped me to turn to my mile-long list of things to do instead of automatically turning to food. I try very hard to eat only when I am relatively happy and calm—not procrastinating, not upset, and not angry. Do not turn to food for comfort; again, it is the problem, not the solution.

Remember, no one is perfect, and if we can live lean 80 percent of the time, we're doing okay. When all else fails, have a legal binge. Eat from my safe list only and allow yourself to have extra if you need it. Giving yourself permission to binge will relieve stress and remove that urge.

> **THE MOST IMPORTANT THING, and I cannot stress it enough, is to learn to forgive yourself if you cheat.** Of all the strategies in this book, this, most of all, is the one thing I want to leave with you. Be confident that you can make this change, so pick yourself up as quickly as possible, brush yourself off, and start fresh right now. Do not wait until tomorrow, Monday, or the New Year.
>
> Because you drink a protein shake every day, you offset those not-so-perfect calories we all eat from time to time. Remember, protein shakes boost your metabolism by 25 percent and block cortisol, the stress hormone, from rising. If you have been following the plan, your metabolism will be revved up and in high gear. *The Metabolism Solution* takes into account that there will be bad days. Simply get right back on the plan and continue like nothing happened.

This is the first day of the rest of your life. You will fall, and you will learn to get up faster and forgive yourself. Focus on progress, not perfection.

SEVEN

GOD AND YOUR BODY

So what does God have to do with it? Everything! I could write a book on this subject alone. Every pain or ache we feel is rooted and intertwined with our emotional and spiritual health. What you believe—or don't believe—keeps you stuck where you are and holds you back from taking care of your health and losing weight. I have learned firsthand that not being able to lose weight has much deeper roots than a slow metabolism.

I now understand that I have to take care of myself, no matter what I'm feeling or experiencing. There is no excuse for not taking care of yourself. Food and emotion used to go hand in hand for me, but I had to learn to stop eating every time I felt an emotion I didn't like. I had to learn to accept and let go of old hurts and fresh wounds, perceived and actual, before I could get a handle on my eating habits and over-exercising. I needed to remember that I had God's love and faith in Him to guide me down the right path. Feelings are very powerful. Any medical doctor will agree that emotions can influence your health—and waistline. And faith has the greatest influence of all.

NOTHING IS MORE IMPORTANT THAN YOUR RELATIONSHIP WITH GOD

If you are serious about changing your body, you need to be serious about working on your relationship with God. I firmly believe that. Only with faith can you get rid of whatever baggage you are carrying or whatever behavior is holding you back. Repressing feelings or denying them won't work. Change starts on the inside. This isn't just about feeling better, losing weight, getting fit. This is much deeper and far greater. This will turn your life around.

- The *only* one you need to please is God.
- The *only* approval you need is from God.
- Listen *only* to what God has to say to you and about you and meditate on this every day:

You are beautiful, precious, courageous, strong.
You are smart, funny, and kind.
You are unique and worthy of love and affection.
You are healthy and vibrant and strong beyond earthly understanding.
You are God's child and your worth surpasses all earthly things.
He loves and adores you.
It is because of Him that you can change your personal circumstance.
It is because of Him that you can change the world.

Are you eating too much to mask a pain, to fill a hole in your heart? Are you happy? A therapist once asked me that particular question, and I struggled to answer it. Outwardly, I'm sure I appeared quite bubbly. I had everything: I had reached my goal weight, I married a loving man and had two beautiful children, we had a nice house complete with four dogs, and my career was going in the direction I wanted. Yet inside, I felt empty. And I couldn't explain why. I still had that emptiness and loneliness inside me from days that weren't so good.

> **YOU CAN'T BE PHYSICALLY FIT UNLESS YOU'RE SPIRITUALLY FIT.**

Again I put the question to you: Are you happy? Do you feel good every day? Are you satisfied with the life you are living? If you had to stop and think about your answer, then you most likely are not happy. It is time to take off the limits you have put on God and let Him into your life. Stop making excuses; trade your negative attitude for a positive one and open your mind as well as your heart. Believe you can be happy and healthy. Have faith. Make the choice to let God in.

The most important decision of your life is to place God in the center of it so that He can guide you to that happy place. Maybe you're already a believer and feel you do this. But has your work, family, or stress over health issues become the center of your thoughts every day? Are you obsessed with spending too much time in the gym or worrying about what you can and cannot eat? Is God in second place with you?

Becoming physically fit did not bring me happiness; it was only half the battle. I needed to become spiritually fit as well. Likewise, becoming spiritually fit (did you know that one in three Christians is overweight?) is only halfway to happiness without the physical component. During my days with Dr. Hatfield and his research studies, I worked with a wide range of bodybuilders and weightlifters. These strong men amazed me. They were able to do things that seemed to defy human understanding, lifting several times their own body

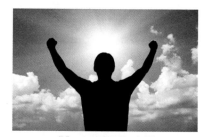

You are God's child

weight. They had faith—and not only in themselves. This group had faith in God. Being physically fit and taking care of the body God gave you is your responsibility; it is another way of worshiping Him. It is your duty and privilege to protect your health.

Coming to this understanding was one of the hardest journeys I've ever been on. I always considered myself a solid Christian woman; but after much, much contemplation, I found that I had started to rely on food more than God. Food became my go-to source whenever anything good or bad happened. I was constantly asking myself, "Why shouldn't I eat this? Why can't I eat that?" I indulged myself. There's a word for you: indulgence. Look it up. It means "unrestrained action." My indulgence was eating. I was seeking pleasure in eating that I did not have in my life. This "pleasure" became unrestrained action and a problem in and of itself. The more I ate to feel better, the more weight I gained. Thus, my initial solution was now most definitely an additional problem. Just as I was, you need to be honest about how you rely on food. I was so lost in feeding my pain that I couldn't hear God's voice. God is here with His arms open in love. Crave God the way you crave food. Don't let food become your god. Use God's presence to fill the void and emptiness that food now fills. Don't let food take God's place. Turn to God in times of stress and sadness, and shout, "Thank you, Jesus!" in times of happiness. Practice living a life full of gratitude and watch the miracles that God has in store for you unfold.

> LET GO AND LET GOD—OR BE DRAGGED

STRENGTHENING YOUR FAITH MUSCLES

> FEAR LOOKS DOWN AND WORRY LOOKS AROUND, BUT FAITH ALWAYS LOOKS UP.

A lack of faith. That is where many problems arise. When things aren't going your way, do you ever think to check in with God? Do you ever wonder whether maybe you would be in a better place if you had a little more faith? Too many people spend too much time looking in the wrong direction, searching for answers. Holding onto resentment is holding onto hopelessness, which is the opposite of faith. Faith is being hopeful, optimistic, and enthusiastic even in the worst situations. Faith is believing God will guide you and show you light in your darkest hour. You cannot be truly physically fit without being spiritually fit. I have no doubts about this truth. You are a spiritual being with a human existence. The two cannot be separated. You are only as strong as your weakest muscle. Do your faith muscles support you?

Every issue you face, from health to finances, can be helped by developing a closer relationship with God. Your belief system affects everything you do—including the foods you eat and the way you live your life. If you don't believe something will work, you won't even take the first step. Your beliefs affect every choice you make every day, including whether to take care of yourself or not.

I made the choice. I chose to see good in every situation, especially the worst ones. I have strengthened my faith muscles by reestablishing my relationship with God. Only then did I begin to lose weight. Faith gives me courage and lets me make changes. Think of it this way: Fear looks down and worry looks around, but faith always looks up.

> All things are possible through Christ who strengthens me!
> —Philippians 4:13

With strong faith muscles you can keep God in the center of all things and never let anything get in the way of your relationship with Him, including your health issues, weight gain, or daily problems. With God all things work out for good; He makes all things possible. Putting God first set me free, and it can do the same for you. If you are living your life based on fear, then you are not leading with faith. As your faith muscles get stronger, you'll lead with faith, and fear won't take you off course. Faith gives you clarity.

> **Hate causes a lot of problems in the world, and it's never fixed even one.**
> —*Maya Angelou*

Think back to feelings and food as discussed in the previous chapter. Dysfunctional beliefs and weak spiritual muscles cause you to become dysfunctional and not take care of yourself; the pain gets fed over and over again. You do not need to be angry to heal; you do not resolve resentments with anger. Anger keeps you stuck where you are. It is a key culprit that weakens your faith muscles. If you are ready to heal and get healthy, both physically and spiritually, you have to let go of your anger, say good-bye to resentments, and find your faith.

> **GOD GRANT ME THE SERENITY TO ACCEPT THE THINGS I CAN-NOT CHANGE, THE COURAGE TO CHANGE THE THINGS THAT I CAN, AND THE WISDOM TO KNOW THE DIFFERENCE.**

Meditation is the exercise needed to strengthen your faith muscles. You might think it different from prayer, you might not. Meditation is a contemplation or thought upon which you reflect. When you meditate on positive things such as God's promises, you will feel good. If you continue to obsess about your problems, you will feel bad, and it will be harder to turn your thoughts around as God's voice gets dimmer. Finding faith is finding optimism, a belief that in God all things will work out. Things happen for reasons you may not be able to understand, and faith helps you get through them.

Faith brings clarity. Faith helps you accept the things you cannot change, but more importantly, faith gives you the wisdom to know the difference between what you need to accept and what you can change. Remember, acceptance is not resignation; acceptance is accepting what is real and not being resentful about it.

To begin to find this clarity, to strengthen your faith muscles, understand this:

> God runs the show.
> God calls the shots.
> All we have to do is show up.
> Don't give away God's power to a diagnosis, a divorce, or any other negative situation.

Give it to God.

We are all God's children, and He loves us all equally and unconditionally.

> **Do you not know that your body is a temple of the Holy Spirit who is in you, whom you have from God, and that you are not your own? For you have been bought with a price. Therefore, glorify God in your body.**
> *—1 Corinthians 6:19*

Think about it. There is always someone out there who is in your corner. You are never alone. Accept this. Use these words as a meditation. Another thought to meditate on: What is God's role in your life? Do you realize the part He plays? Do you grasp how much He loves you? Listen only to what God has to say about you, and He thinks very highly of you. Regardless of who you think you are or how you feel, you are the child of the Most High God who is powerful and strong. It is because of Him that you have the ability to change the world and your circumstances (all of them) forever.

God loves you, He adores you, and He created you to be fearless and courageous so that you can go strengthen your spiritual muscles. Find that person who may be buried under 40 pounds of excess weight or under that diagnosis that is holding you down or under any fear that has been paralyzing you and clouding your thinking. Tap into the God source and release that person you were created to be. It's your responsibility to set that person free.

Once you practice these meditation exercises, you will begin to see His work in your life and begin to remove the obstacles that keep you from seeing God's grace. You will strengthen your faith muscles.

> The only being you need to please is God.
> The only approval you ever need is God's.

Any other voices that are telling you bad things about yourself are nothing more than your spiritual muscles begging you to give them a workout. Go back to the basic meditations listed here as many times as it takes, until you feel better or see the change you are waiting for.

For every problem, God has a solution. Take it to God. Give everything to God: Worry about nothing and pray about everything. Prayer is heavenly intervention and gives God your permission for Him to step in. In order to be healthy spiritually, we need to pray every day.

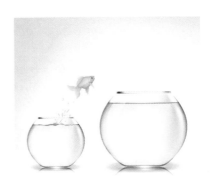

Faith frees you from limitations

If you are stuck and just cannot lose weight or change your circumstances, you need to ask yourself: What are you meditating on every day? Your own problems? Or our God's solutions? We all meditate every day without even knowing it. If you meditate on gratitude, you feel grateful; if you meditate on how bad your problems are, you'll always see your life through your problems, and you won't be able to see clearly. Faith gives you clarity.

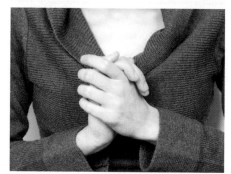

Strengthen your faith muscles with prayer

The bottom line? Most people meditate on pain, which causes them to relive pain, often from a very long time ago. Why do they—and why do you—continue to feel pain from things that happened so long ago? Pain can actually serve a very productive purpose. Its appearance, physical and spiritual, alerts you to the need to address something. Unfortunately, if your faith muscles are not strong enough, the pain won't fulfill its productive role; instead, it will drag you down.

What course of action is open to you when you know you have faith muscles weakened by anger and resentment? Find the truth about yourself. Listening to truths about yourself is not easy; it's downright hard. But to process the feelings and ultimately feel God's love, you need to listen to those truths.

Now that you've done the basics with meditation, you can further strengthen your faith muscles with prayer. Spend quiet time with God every day. I know how difficult this can be in our busy world, so here is a way to begin praying:

QUIET TIME WITH GOD TO STRENGTHEN YOUR FAITH MUSCLES

- *Be alone with God and willingly bring your entire self to Him.*
- *Allow your mind to settle so your soul can emerge. Breathe in and out slowly and focus on your breathing until you feel relaxed.*
- *Recognize that God is as near as your own breath. If you are holding your breath or not exhaling, you are blocking God from entering.*
- *Hear God calling, "Come away with Me to rest a while."*
- *Is there anything that is hurting you or that you're struggling with these days? What is it that you have been holding onto? Have you lost your perspective?*
- *Allow it to come to the surface, whether it seems big or small—God will guide you through it so you can relax.*
- *Whatever feelings rise to the surface (you will need time to become aware of some of them), know that you are not alone. You are in the presence of the One who loves you.*

- *Trust your deepest feelings and thoughts to God.*
- *Is there something you're feeling stressed about lately? Is something bothering you physically or spiritually? Ask God what you need to see. Perhaps you are grateful and need to express gratitude? God loves thankfulness.*
- *Let it rise to the surface without judging. Bask in the goodness of God instead of letting your feelings override God's grace.*
- *When your quiet time with God is over, carry the sense of being alone with God with you into your day.*
- *When you begin to feel stressed, repeat this process as often as needed.*

FOR BEST RESULTS: Practice these steps three times each day. Find a quiet place where you will not be interrupted. I suggest doing your spiritual workout first thing in the morning before anyone is up. That's what Jesus did.

> **...Take time and trouble to keep yourself spiritually fit. Bodily fitness has limited value, but spiritual fitness is of unlimited value, for it holds promise both for this present life and for the life to come.**
> —*1 Timothy 4:7-8*

Remember to focus on your breathing; breathe in and out as slowly as you can. If you are harried and stressed, gently slow down your breathing. Inhale deeply and exhale as slowly as possible in order to relax your body. Tell your body to wilt as you slowly exhale (especially the tense, tight muscles) so you're totally relaxed and open to receiving. Take your time and take as many deep "cleansing" breaths as you need to feel relaxed. A cleansing breath is when you exhale hard and visualize any ache or pain you have as well as any negative thoughts leaving your body. Each time you exhale, visualize all of your stress leaving and God taking it to handle for you.

When my mind races, I pray the serenity prayer: "God grant me the serenity to accept the things I cannot change, the courage to change the things that I can, and the wisdom to know the difference."

I struggle with learning how to love, how to forgive, and how to nurture myself. I never miss a weight workout or a serving of broccoli anymore, but sometimes I miss my quiet prayer or meditation. I miss God's voice because I cannot hear it when I'm moving at 100 miles an hour. I need to be slowed down enough to hear His voice, and if I'm in a loving place with myself, I can receive His help. Did you follow that? I am not always in a loving place with myself, and that's why I don't eat clean or take care of my body by working out. Not being in a loving place with myself means, more importantly, that I am not going to be open to receiving God's healing. If I don't love myself, I won't feel that I am worthy; and if I don't believe I am worthy, I most likely will never take the proper steps to reach my goals.

Do you now see how belief and faith have everything to do with outcomes? If you are walking around

30, 50, or 100 pounds or more overweight, you are letting the world know that you don't love yourself and do not take care of yourself, inside and out.

Are you ready to radically transform your life, not just your body? Remove any and all limitations you have placed on God and allow Him to do His work. He wants to bless you with your heart's desires no matter what they are (but especially the physical ones). This spiritually leaner lifestyle also comes with the side effect of abundant peace, joy, and a love that surrounds you, making you feel whole, complete, and loved in ways you've never experienced before.

> **THE 10-SECOND SPIRITUAL DETOX**
> **Ask yourself if there is one thing, event, or person that you can think of that makes your blood boil. Give yourself 10 seconds to think about it and then stop. What came up? Unfortunately, this meditation exercise may not leave you relaxed upon completion, but it will ultimately help you regain your faith. It's important to do it until you can figure out what or who you need to forgive and process those feelings so you can be free from the pain.**

If you're ready, you can surrender all of your stress, anxiety, and health issues simply by following the rules already set in the Bible. *The Metabolism Solution* simply helps you with recipes and exercises that bring God closer to you so you can actually hear His voice and see where He is trying to lead you. Did you know that crazy lifestyles (including over-volunteering at church) can make it difficult to really hear what it is God wants you to hear? Being intimately in touch with God brings an emotional sobriety to your life. When you aren't eating right or working out or resting enough or spending enough time alone with God so He can talk to you directly, you are "emotionally drunk." You cannot hear God's voice the way you need to in order to make necessary physical, mental, or lifestyle changes that will heal your life and not just your body. Do the 10-Second Spiritual Detox Exercise described previously. It's not easy (to say the least) to face unpleasant feelings. And food, especially those sugar-laden and unhealthy foods which give you a "sugar high," can stifle your feelings. Try eating clean for a week and then doing this meditation. It holds the secret to your success.

CLEANSING FOR CLARITY

Sometimes no matter how hard you might try to focus on the good things, all you can see is the bad. Fasting can really help with this. All religions include fasting, and some have upheld the tradition for centuries. Fasting is more than just not eating meat on Fridays. Fasting is a way to leave behind the physical, focus on the spiritual, and become closer to God. My pastor, Frank Santora, put it this way: "Fasting empowers us to progress rapidly toward the heart of God. When we deny our flesh, our spirit becomes more sensitive to the voice of God. Any time we deny our flesh, our spiritual antennae become more sensitive to God's voice."

His fellow pastor, Rich Perez, added, "Fasting allows us to remove the mindset of self-centeredness and allows us to become totally dependent on our Creator, rather than our own resources and self. It removes our dependency upon all things that block our sensitivity to our spirit."

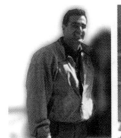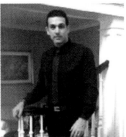

Pastor Frank – Lost 67 Pounds!
Real People, Real Results

I fly a lot for various appearances, and on one flight I was lucky enough to sit next to a rabbi with whom I had a wonderful discussion about God. We touched upon fasting, and Rabbi Shmuly concurred with these two pastors. "There is no need to eat when we are focused on God. By fasting, we rise above the everyday and live on a higher spiritual plane. Fasting creates a euphoria that energizes us."

> **IF YOU WAN-NA GET RID OF THE PUDGE, YOU GOTTA LET GO OF THE GRUDGE. FASTING AND GIVING IT TO GOD ARE THE SOLUTION.**

Jesus fasted to hear and understand God's voice and His directions for His life. So should we.

For me, fasting is a life-changing experience. At the beginning of my weight loss journey, I specifically fasted or abstained from the foods I was addicted to—carbohydrates, cheese, and processed foods. I stopped those instant-gratification food fixes. Instead of obsessing over what I ate, I was free to focus on life and what God wanted for me. Elements of this plan came to me at those times, and more importantly came my deeper feeling of God's love.

Moses fasted for 40 days. Jesus fasted for 40 days. Fasting helps bring us back to God, to family, to love. There is no instant gratification in fasting; there is only the deep and lasting satisfaction that comes from a connection to God.

My decades of training and helping others reach their weight loss goals has taught me that people do better on a highly structured plan, even when fasting. And remember, fasting doesn't always have to be about food. You can fast from exercise if you're an over-exerciser (just walk every day for health) and see your life fall into proper perspective. *The Metabolism Solution* has helped me not only lose weight and keep it off, but it has also helped me stay directly connected to God. I hear His voice clearly without interference. When I fall off the fast, off my plan, all the anxiety and stinking thinking come back tenfold.

WWJD. I LIVE BY THE SAYING "WHAT WOULD JESUS DO?" BUT HAVE YOU EVER WONDERED WHAT JESUS DID TO KEEP HIMSELF FED AND FIT? WHAT DID JESUS DO? HAVE YOU EVER GIVEN A THOUGHT TO HOW MUCH AND HOW FAR JESUS MUST HAVE WALKED? JESUS WORSHIPPED BY TAKING CARE OF HIS BODY. WE ARE SUPPOSED TO IMITATE HIM. DO YOU?

YES, JESUS NEVER HAD TO WORRY ABOUT ALL THE SNACK FOOD CHOICES WE FACE TODAY, AND HE DIDN'T HAVE THE CONVENIENCE OF AUTOMOBILES. FOODS WERE OFTEN SIMPLER, CLEANER. PHYSICAL LABOR AND HAVING TO WALK EVERYWHERE KEPT PEOPLE FIT. WE CAN ALL BECOME LIKE CHRIST—BY FOLLOWING THE OVERALL STYLE OF LIFE HE CHOSE FOR HIMSELF. PRAYER, MEDITATION ON GOD'S WORD, AND FASTING KEPT JESUS CLOSE TO GOD. IF WE HAVE FAITH IN CHRIST, WE MUST BELIEVE HE KNEW HOW TO LIVE.

JESUS ATE FROM THE EARTH. HE ATE VEGETABLES AND FISH AND SMALL AMOUNTS OF LEAN MEATS. OF COURSE HE ATE FIGS AND NUTS, AND HE SIPPED ON WINE (SIPPED IS THE POINT). HE WALKED EVERYWHERE SO HE WAS CONDITIONED. JESUS ATE DINNER EARLY WHEN THE SUN WAS GOING DOWN AND WOKE UP EARLY AT SUNRISE. THERE IS MUCH MORE TO LEARN FROM THE BEST TEACHER THAT EVER WAS THAN YOU THINK.

WHEN IN DOUBT, ASK YOURSELF: WHAT DID JESUS DO?

The Metabolism Solution provides you with a plan that includes intermittent fasting to rev up your metabolism (full-on fasting would slow down your metabolism) and not hurt your weight loss goals the way other fasts can. No, I don't propose you go without food and water for days at a time, but I do see great benefit in my 48-hour Metabolic-Boosting Fast. When I've fallen off my plan and indulged in my favorite guilty food pleasure, had a special dinner night out where I didn't eat cleanly, or am feeling out of sorts with the world around me and need to reconnect with God, a fast gets me back on track.

Any situation can be helped if you believe it can be. So why don't you believe you can lose weight? Are you lacking confidence? Worried? Worry is a lack of faith in God; replace your worry with faith in God. When struggling with health or financial issues or with personal problems that never seem to end, it becomes increasingly harder to hear God's voice. It's not impossible to hear God; you just have to work harder.

BELIEVING AND DOING WHATEVER IT TAKES

Are you willing to do whatever it takes? Are you willing to do whatever needs to be done for as long as it takes? Your body is not your god. Your scale is not your god. Food is not your god. Seek God the way you seek a good meal, and you'll never be hungry again.

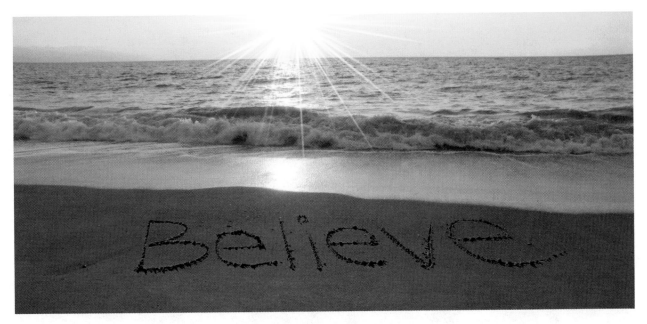

Replace your worry with belief in God

If there were a red button that you could push to make losing weight and getting in shape faster and easier, would you push it? Guess what? You just did by reading this book.

The Metabolism Solution is the answer to your weight loss problems. Are you ready for life-changing, radical transformations? Are you ready for vibrant health and vitality? All you have to lose is the extra weight. Unlike other programs, *The Metabolism Solution* is guaranteed to work if you work it—or I'll gladly refund your misery. You have to believe, or you'll never even start. You have what it takes. I know you do. God is on your side, so how can you fail? Get ready for the new, leaner, happier, and more vibrant you.

Start today!

METABOLISM SOLUTION CHEAT SHEETS

I am so confident that you will find success with weight loss, better health and vitality, and overall fitness with *The Metabolism Solution*. I created this plan with YOU in mind. I want to you experience the success that so many of my clients have achieved. More than anything else, I want you to discover the person that God created you to be—physically, emotionally, and spiritually.

I happen to agree wholeheartedly with the idea that if you fail to plan, you plan to fail. One way to guarantee success on this program is to prepare. Get to the grocery store and buy the healthy, clean food on the plan. Go out and buy yourself a pair (or two!) of dumbbells for your Metabolic Workout. Write out what you plan to eat each day BEFORE the week begins, or at least have a basic framework in mind.

With all that in mind, I've created this Resource Section for you to use as your go-to jumping off point. Confused about what you can and can't eat? Check out the Meal Plan, Food Lists, and Metabolic Cleanse guides. Want a simple checklist of what to buy at the grocery store? Check out the Shopping List. Not sure what workouts to do each day? Simply consult the Workouts page.

Everything has been mapped out for you—all you have to do is begin! Are you ready? Let's do this.

YOUR GOAL WEIGHT X 10 = TOTAL CALORIES FOR THE DAY

Step one is to figure out your daily calorie goal. Use the formula above to calculate your total calorie intake for each day. Other suggestions to keep in mind on *The Metabolism Solution*:

1. Start your day with whey to boost your metabolism by 25 percent. Within one hour of waking, drink a whey-based protein shake. The best shakes have about 155 calories; low carb—under 20 grams; low fat—less than 5 grams; and 20-24 grams of protein. For the best weight loss results, stay with whey protein—no soy, pea or potato protein. Always look for the highest quality whey protein from a reputable source.
2. Limit fat. Keep your daily fat intake to 15 grams max for women and 20 grams max for men and teens. Choose only essential fats.
3. Be careful with carbs. Consume non-vegetable carbohydrates (if you insist on eating them) before 3:00 p.m. If you're losing too slowly, drop carbs completely (vegetables do not count). Keep your non-vegetable carbs under 75 grams per day.
4. Power your metabolism with protein. Eat 25 grams of lean protein (see list) per meal.
5. Read labels to be lean. Check calorie counts and weigh and measure everything or look it

up in a calorie book. This one simple step can make or break your weight loss.

6. Water for weight loss. Drink half your body weight in ounces of water daily. That's 8 to 10 8-oz. glasses a day—minimum.

7. Snack slim. Keep snacks at 100 calories or less. Better yet, choose veggies or fruit.

8. Timing is everything. Keep a minimum of three hours between meals. If you eat in between, your body cannot digest the food and will store it as fat. This could also cause insulin to rise and slow down all the metabolic boosting you've been working so hard on.

9. Food is only half your day. Eat all your meals in a 12-hour window (7:00 a.m. to 7:00 p.m., for example).

10. Get HUNGRY! Hunger is a good sign. It means your body is about to burn fat. The feeling will dissipate. You don't need to instantly gratify every food craving. Find another way to entertain yourself—change a thought and move muscle, anything BUT succumb to eating again. You will not be literally starving. It was a pivotal moment for me when I learned it was okay to be hungry. Hunger is a sign your body is about to start burning fat. Don't let hunger pangs scare you.

METABOLIC BOOSTING FOOD LIST

These are your go-to foods to keep your metabolism fired up on all cylinders. If it's not on the list, don't eat it! Aim to stick to this list 100%, but don't get discouraged if you slip up. Just have a metabolic-boosting protein shake and get right back on the plan. When you eat these foods, you are priming your body for ultimate calorie burning, fat burning and revving of your metabolism. You will feel better, look better, and experience vibrant health. I promise you!

Proteins (Three to Four Per Day)

High-quality Whey Protein Shake (2 per day max.)
Protein Bar (2 per day max.)
Egg Whites (3 to 4)
Scrod/Cod, 4 oz.
Flounder, 4 oz.
Haddock, 4 oz.
Halibut, 4 oz.
Scallops, 4 oz.
Orange Roughy, 4 oz.
Grouper, 4 oz.
Tilapia, 4 oz.
Shrimp, 4 oz. (shelled)
Sea Bass, 4 oz.
Snapper, 4 oz. (all)
Mussels, 4 oz.
Chicken Breast, 3 oz. (no skin)

Nonfat Cottage Cheese, ½ cup
Tuna, Fresh or Canned, 3 oz.
Mahi-Mahi, 4 oz.
Clams, 4 oz.
Mussels, 4 oz.
Oysters, 5 oz.
Crab, 4 oz.
Lobster, 1½ lbs. (whole)
Calamari, 4-5 oz.
Salmon, 4 oz.
Swordfish, 4 oz.
Sashimi, 4 oz.
Sardines, 3 oz.
Herring, 4 oz.
Trout/Rainbow Trout, 4 oz.
Sashimi, 4 oz.
Turkey Breast, 3 oz. (no skin)

Vegetables (Ten Servings Per Day)

These are your new best friends! They will melt away the fat with their inherent thermogenic properties. Experiment with the recipes in the book and don't be afraid to try new foods. Your body—and your waistline—will thank you.

Alfalfa Sprouts
Asparagus
Broccoflower
Broccoli
Brussel Sprouts
Cabbage (all types)
Carrots
Cauliflower
Celery

Collard Greens
Cucumbers
Eggplant
Escarole
Green Beans
Kale
Lettuce (all types; serving is 3 cups)
Onion

Radishes
Spinach
Tomato Juice (4 oz.)
Tomatoes
Yellow Beans
Yellow Squash
Wax Beans
Zucchini

Low-Sugar Fruits (Two Per Day)

High in enzymes and minerals, fruit is nature's natural cleanser. Enjoy two fruits per day maximum. A portion is one half cup or as noted. Fresh or frozen (without added sugar) is fine. Always choose organic.

Apple (Granny Smith is best), 1 small
Berries (Blueberries, Blackberries), 1 cup
Cantaloupe and ALL Melons, ½ cup
Grapefruit, ½ small or ½ cup
Kiwi, 1 small
Cherries, 10 large
Raspberries, 1 cup
Strawberries, 1 cup
Oranges, 1 small
Nectarines, 1 small
Peaches, 1 small
Pears, 1 small
Plums, 2 medium

"Healthy" Carbs (Limit These)

While these foods may be considered healthy, they also spike blood sugar levels, which slows the weight loss process. The bottom line—the fewer carbs you eat, the faster you will lose weight. I'm not preaching 100 percent carb avoidance here, but when you are losing weight, you need to focus on eating carbs that are BETTER at boosting metabolism, aka vegetables! I also know that we all live in the real world and most of us will eat out at times, choosing snacks that are off-plan, and falling into the "carb pit." Aiming to eat less of the following carbs is best for melting belly fat faster.

All Bran (½ cup)
Barley (½ cup)
Beans – *Black, Fava, Garbanzo, Kidney, Lentils, Lima, Northern, Pinto, Red, Soy, White* (2 tablespoons)
Popcorn (air popped, 3 cups)
Corn (½ cup)
Fiber One Cereal (½ cup)
Oatmeal (slow cooking, ½ cup)
Parsnips (½ cup)
Pasta (½ cup)
Brown or Wild Rice (½ cup)
Rice Bran (½ cup)
Sweet Potato (½ cup)
Wasa Light (1 piece)
Whole Grain Breads (1 oz.)
Winter Squash (all varieties, ½ cup)

Condiments

No fats, no sauces, no cheeses! You need to watch the fat and sugar content in every product you buy. Better yet, make your own salad dressings and sauces using the recipes in this book.

Vinegar – there are so many tasty, healthy varieties
Low-sodium, low-fat broths
Pepper
Spices: basil, cayenne, cinnamon, garlic, ginger, oregano, turmeric, etc.
NoSalt
Mrs. Dash Seasoning

Legal Snacks List

Air-Popped Popcorn, 3 cups (60 calories)
Clear Broth Soup
Fudgsicles (25 to 40 calories)
Garden Salad
Green Apple, 1 small
Sugarless gum
Sugar-Free Candy, 2 pieces
Sugar Free Gelatin
Sugar-Free Popsicles (15 to 25 calories)
Tomato Juice
Tootsie Roll Pop (25 calories)

METABOLISM SOLUTION MEAL PLAN

This is the base plan that you can stick with for the rest of your life. Starting your day with a whey protein shake makes all the difference. This one drink revs up your metabolism for the rest of the day. If you just replace your usual breakfast with a whey protein shake, you'll see a difference; but if you follow *The Metabolism Solution*, you'll see change. Once the weight begins to come off, you can replace your lunchtime shake with vegetables and a lean protein. You'll find plenty of satisfying and filling foods to choose from within these pages and some metabolism-revving recipes as well. If you stop losing weight or slow down, go back to a shake for lunch. Give it a try; you have nothing to lose but the pounds.

BREAKFAST
- Whey protein shake made with water or protein bar
- Black coffee or tea

SNACK
- Small apple

LUNCH
- Whey protein shake made with water or protein bar
- (or lean protein and vegetables once weight starts coming off)

SNACK
- Small apple or any fruit from low-sugar fruits or legal snacks lists

DINNER
- Choose one serving of any lean protein from the list and a large salad with a minimum of five servings of vegetables from the list

SNACK
- Anything from the legal snacks list (nothing to eat after 8:00 p.m.)

During the Metabolic Cleanse, you will be following the meal plan on the previous page but limiting your lunch to ONLY the protein shake made with water.

METABOLIC-BOOSTING CLEANSE

You will use this cleanse to kick start your Metabolism Solution Eating Plan and get your body revved up and ready to lose weight. You can also go back to this cleanse any time you hit a plateau or just need to "reset" your body.

BREAKFAST
- Whey protein shake
- Multivitamin to provide nutrients and energy
- Green tea as desired throughout day

LUNCH
- Whey protein shake
- Omega-3 supplement to curb cravings (can use as a snack replacement if required)

DINNER
- Green vegetables (5 ½-cup servings) and white fish (1 serving)
- 2 raspberry ketone capsules

BEDTIME
- Melatonin supplement to provide restful and revitalizing sleep

Drink at least half your body weight in ounces of water throughout the day to cleanse and rid your body of toxins!

EXERCISE ON THE METABOLISM SOLUTION

Eating right is so important on *The Metabolism Solution*, but exercise goes hand in hand with your healthy eating plan. For your mental and physical health, you absolutely need to move every day. I recommend doing a Metabolic Core Walk, which I outline in chapter five. You will need to start working with dumbbells—start with a weight you are comfortable with and can safely perform 12-15 reps with proper form—to see the fastest results and build up your bones. Twenty minutes a week can halt osteoporosis! Use my Metabolic Workout in chapter five as the foundation for your strength training routine.

Cardiovascular Exercise

- Start with walking or stationary biking 20 minutes a day, then work up to 60 minutes, 5 times a week.
  * Work up to the point where you can walk 5 miles or bike 15-18 miles in 60 minutes.
  * You can break up your walking/biking into 20-minute increments.

Metabolic Workout (three times a week)

- Deep Squat to Front Raise
- Stiff Leg Dead Lift
- Side Lunge with Arm Curl
- Front Lunge with Side Raise
- Bent Over Dumbbell Row in Lunge Position
- Tricep Dip
- Pushups
- Lying Rear Fly
- Side Core Raise
- Plank

Visit www.lynfit.com for downloadable videos and other fitness tips.

Shopping List

The whole point of this shopping list is for you to have everything you need to eat available to you so that you can plan to succeed. When that hungry feeling hits (and it invariably will), you need to have all of your healthy-eating arsenal ready to help you avoid temptation and ensure your success.

Most of your eating will be concentrated on vegetables and lean white protein, such as white fish and egg whites. Check out my recipes and add ingredients that you want to try to this list! I recommend that you start off without the whole grain breads, rice, and pastas that are listed on the "Healthy Carbs" List until you get close to your goal weight. While these can be incorporated later, they will only slow your weight loss in the beginning.

Protein (Meat, Fish, and Dairy Departments)

- Several varieties of white fish, fresh or flash frozen (haddock, tilapia, halibut, shrimp, etc.)
- Boneless, skinless chicken breast
- Turkey breast
- Tuna—fresh, frozen, or canned in water
- Low-fat red meat, such as bison (if available)
- Nonfat cottage cheese
- Egg whites or egg substitute like Egg Beaters

Produce Department

- Lots of leafy greens (lettuce, collards, escarole, kale, spinach, etc.)
- Asparagus
- Berries (blueberries, blackberries, strawberries, cherries)
- Broccoli & broccoflower
- Brussels sprouts
- Cauliflower
- Cabbage
- Celery
- Carrots
- Cucumber
- Eggplant
- Granny Smith apples
- Grapefruit

- Green, yellow, and wax beans
- Kiwi
- Onion
- Nectarines
- Peaches
- Pears
- Plums
- Radishes
- Squash
- Zucchini

Pantry

- Vinegar (Apple cider, balsamic, red wine)
- Low-sodium chicken and/or vegetable broth
- Sugar-free Jell-O gelatin
- Popcorn kernels to air pop
- Spices
- Pepper
- NoSalt or other salt substitute like Mrs. Dash
- Sugar-free candy

Supplements and Protein Shakes/Bars*

- High-quality whey protein shakes
- Protein bars (watch sugar and carb content)

My Top Ten "Superstar Supplements" List**

1. Raspberry ketones
2. Cocoa bean powder
3. Green tea
4. Forskolin
5. Banaba leaf
6. Gugglesterones
7. White kidney bean extract
8. Melatonin
9. Omega-3
10. Vitamin D

*Be sure to read and follow labels

Optional:

A daily Multivitamin

Cleansing supplement

**Visit my website at www.lynfit.com for a variety of supplements and products to support your journey on *The Metabolism Solution*.

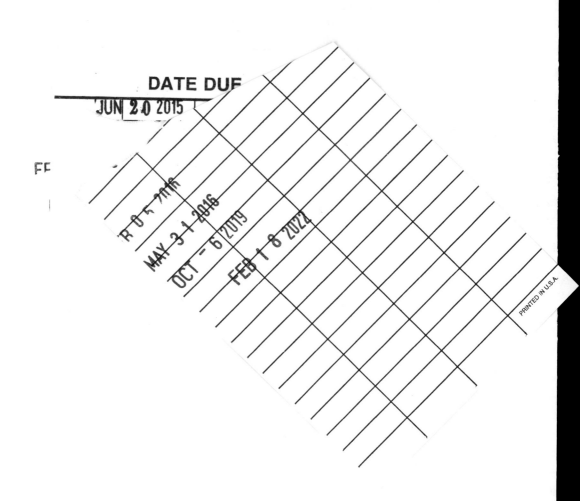

DATE DUE

JUN 2 0 2015

FE

R 0 5 2016

MAY 3 1 2016

OCT - 6 2019

FEB 1 8 2022